A Systems Approach To Social And Organizational Planning.

Cure For The Mess In Health Care?

Gerrit Van Wyk

Trafford Publishing
Victoria, BC

© Copyright 2003 Gerrit Van Wyk. All rights reserved.

No part of this publication may be reproduced, stored in a retrieval system, or transmitted, in any form or by any means, electronic, mechanical, photocopying, recording, or otherwise, without the written prior permission of the author.

Illustrator: Johann Wessels — www.johannwessels.com

Note for Librarians: a cataloguing record for this book that includes Dewey Classification and US Library of Congress numbers is available from the National Library of Canada. The complete cataloguing record can be obtained from the National Library s online database at:
www.nlc-bnc.ca/amicus/index-e.html

ISBN 1-4120-1390-9

TRAFFORD

This book was published on-demand in cooperation with Trafford Publishing.
On-demand publishing is a unique process and service of making a book available for retail sale to the public taking advantage of on-demand manufacturing and Internet marketing. On-demand publishing includes promotions, retail sales, manufacturing, order fulfilment, accounting and collecting royalties on behalf of the author.

Suite 6E, 2333 Government St., Victoria, B.C. V8T 4P4, CANADA
Phone   250-383-6864   Toll-free   1-888-232-4444 (Canada & US)
Fax   250-383-6804   E-mail   sales@trafford.com
Web site www.trafford.com TRAFFORD PUBLISHING IS A DIVISION OF TRAFFORD HOLDINGS LTD.
Trafford Catalogue #03-1768   www.trafford.com/robots/03-1768.html
10   9   8   7   6   5   4   3   2

Contents

ILLUSTRATIONS — VI

TABLES — VII

PREFACE — 1

INTRODUCTION: WHY SHOULD I USE SYSTEMS THINKING TO PLAN? — 3

PART 1: SYSTEMS THINKING — 8

CHAPTER 1: AN ARCHAEOLOGY OF SYSTEMS AND RELATED THINKING — 9

GENERAL SYSTEMS THEORY — 11
CYBERNETICS — 12
GENERAL LIVING SYSTEMS THEORY — 12
HARD SYSTEMS — 13
SOFT SYSTEMS — 14
SYSTEMS METHODOLOGIES — 15
STUDIES OF COMPLEXITY, CHAOS AND NON-LINEARITY — 18

CHAPTER 2: SYSTEMS CONCEPTS — 21

DEFINITION OF A SYSTEM — 23

i

STRUCTURE	25
PROCESS	25
FUNCTION	28
STABILITY	28
SUMMARY	30
LIVING SYSTEMS	31

CHAPTER 3: HUMAN ACTIVITY SYSTEMS　　34

STABILITY	35
VICKERS' MODEL OF SOCIAL INTERACTION	38
RESPONSIBILITY AND NORMS	39
MODERN MAN	40
MODELS OF ORGANIZATION	42
CONTROL	44
CAUSALITY IN COMPLEX SYSTEMS	45
POWER INTERACTIONS	49
TYPES OF POWER	50
THE POWER MOTIVE	51
WHO HOLDS POWER?	53
THE ACQUISITION OF POWER	54
ETHICAL POWER	55
PURPOSEFUL BEHAVIOR	57
REASON	58

CHAPTER 4: KNOWLEDGE ABOUT COMPLEX PHENOMENA　　60

WHAT IS KNOWLEDGE?	60
LEARNING: ALTERING KNOWLEDGE	61
MIND MAPS: SHARED KNOWLEDGE	64
IMAGE OF SELF	64
RESISTANCE TO CHANGE	65
PERFECTION OF IMAGE	65
SHARED IMAGES	65
FACT NETS: ORGANIZED KNOWLEDGE	67
KNOWLEDGE IN DECISION-MAKING	68

CHAPTER 5: KNOWLEDGE AND INQUIRY. C WEST CHURCHMAN'S SYSTEMS PHILOSOPHY — 73

THE PHILOSOPHICAL FRAMEWORK — **76**
RATIONALISM — 77
EMPIRICISM — 78
CRITICISM — 79
SPECULATIVE METHOD — 80
POSITIVISTIC METHOD — 80
PRAGMATISM — 81
SUMMARY — 83
CHURCHMAN'S DESIGN OF INQUIRING SYSTEMS — **84**
DESIGN AND INQUIRY — 84
WHOLE SYSTEMS AND GOAL SEEKING — 85
A THEORY OF KNOWLEDGE — 86
SUMMARY — 97
THE SYSTEMS APPROACH — **98**
THE SYSTEMS VIEW — 98
LOGIC — 103
METHODOLOGY — 104
ETHICS — 110
INTERPRETATION — 112
CONCLUSION — 114

PART 2: A SYSTEMS APPROACH TO HEALTH CARE PLANNING — 115

INTRODUCTION — 116

CHAPTER 6: THE PROBLEM SITUATION. HEALTH CARE IS A MESS — 119

THE PROBLEM SITUATION — **119**
STRUCTURE — **120**
BUDGETARY CONSTRAINTS — 120
OVER SUPPLY OF PHYSICIANS — 121
UNLIMITED PATIENT DEMAND — 122

HIGH TECHNOLOGY HOSPITAL BASED CARE	123
OVER SERVICING	123
THE AGEING POPULATION	124
PROCESS	**125**
FUNCTION AND STABILITY	**128**
INPUT	128
DRAWINGS	129
CONTROLLING THE COST SPIRAL	129
WHAT LESSONS FROM THE MESS?	**141**

CHAPTER 7: AN ARCHAEOLOGY OF THE PROBLEM SITUATION — 144

HISTORY OF THE PATIENT-PHYSICIAN INTERACTION	**144**
PRE-SCIENTIFIC (ANCIENT) ERA	145
SCIENTIFIC ERA	148
TECHNOLOGICAL ERA	151
INFORMATION ERA	154
WORLDVIEW	**154**
THE WORLDVIEW OF HEALTH	155
THE PHYSICIAN	160

CHAPTER 8: THE PATIENT-PHYSICIAN SYSTEM — 163

THE PATIENT-PHYSICIAN SYSTEM	**163**
THE CONSULTATION SYSTEM	**167**
THE CONSULTATION	167
THE DIAGNOSTIC SYSTEM	177
TREATMENT	193
SYNTHESIS	**199**
CONCLUSION	**201**

CHAPTER 9: A SYSTEMS APPROACH TO HEALTH CARE PLANNING — 202

THE PATIENT-PHYSICIAN SYSTEM AS A LEARNING SYSTEM	**203**
A SYSTEMS MODEL OF HEALTH CARE	203
THE HEALTH CARE SYSTEM AS A PURPOSEFUL SYSTEM	**207**
THE PATIENT-PHYSICIAN SYSTEM	208

PHYSICIANS	208
PATIENTS	208
THE PHYSICIAN NETWORK SYSTEM	210
THE HEALTH CARE SYSTEM IN TERMS OF CHURCHMAN'S METHODOLOGY	**215**
CLIENTS (THE SOURCE OF MOTIVATION)	215
PLANNERS (THE SOURCE OF EXPERTISE)	218
THE DECISION MAKER (THE SOURCE OF CONTROL)	221
SYSTEMS PHILOSOPHY (THE SOURCE OF LEGITIMATION)	224
A CHURCHMANIAN APPROACH TO THE DIAGNOSIS-TREATMENT SYSTEM	**227**
SUMMARY	**231**
SYNTHESIS	**232**

CHAPTER 10: THE DECISION SUPPORT SYSTEM — 238

SOFT SYSTEMS METHODOLOGY	**238**
THE DECISION SUPPORT SYSTEM	**240**
APPRECIATION	240
CHURCHMAN'S INQUIRING SYSTEM	240
SYSTEMS METHODOLOGIES	240
LEARNING	243
IMPLEMENTATION AND CHANGE	244
SUMMARY	**245**

EPILOGUE — 246

BIBLIOGRAPHY — 249

INDEX — 265

v

Illustrations

Diagram 1:	A Hierarchy of knowledge...............................	21
Diagram 2:	System viewpoints...	24
Diagram 3:	The transformation of MEI.............................	26
Diagram 4:	Systems perspectives.......................................	30
Diagram 5:	Growth and constraint.....................................	36
Diagram 6:	Feedback...	47
Diagram 7:	Animal populations...	48
Diagram 8:	Complex causal systems..................................	49
Diagram 9:	Power interactions..	51
Diagram 10:	Kolb's learning cycle......................................	62
Diagram 11:	Problem solving...	71
Diagram 12:	Lockean agreement...	89
Diagram 13:	Churchman's learning cycle.........................	105
Diagram 14:	The health care system...................................	116
Diagram 15:	A system dynamics model of the mess in health care	125
Diagram 16:	Balancing funding..	128
Diagram 17:	Health..	155
Diagram 18:	The patient-physician system.......................	165
Diagram 19:	The patient-physician interaction.................	166
Diagram 20:	The diagnostic cycle.......................................	178
Diagram 21:	Medical diagnosis as a learning cycle.........	179
Diagram 22:	Abbreviated diagnosis....................................	180
Diagram 23:	The traditional gatekeeper system................	187
Diagram 24:	The dynamics of the patient-physician interaction....	199
Diagram 25:	The prevalence of illness in society.............	204
Diagram 26:	A systems model of health............................	206
Diagram 27:	The physician network system......................	211
Diagram 28:	Cost effective patient-physician interaction............	232
Diagram 29:	The effect of a systems model on the mess in health care...	235
Diagram 30:	Soft Systems Methodology............................	238
Diagram 31:	The Decision Support System.......................	239
Diagram 32:	Kolb's learning cycle and SSM.....................	242

Tables

Table 1:	Modes of inquiry	31
Table 2:	Social control	41
Table 3:	Purposeful behavior in organizations	42
Table 4:	A comparison of Torbert's and Flood and Jackson's concepts of power	50
Table 5:	A classification of primary error types according to the cognitive stages at which they occur	70
Table 6:	Selection of Family Practitioners	170
Table 7:	Error in decision-making	230
Table 8:	A grouping of problem contexts	241

Preface

Training in the professions rarely includes coursework in the philosophy of science. As a result of this, coming from a profession, I found the transition to systems thinking a difficult one to make. All texts about systems thinking are either of a superficial nature, or assume that the reader has the necessary background to understand the intricacies of the argument. This may result in an erroneous belief, either that the systems approach is simplistic, or that it is too difficult to grasp. In addition, important systems texts, none more so than the work of C West Churchman, are out of print and therefore not readily available or accessible. As a result of this, those who stand most to benefit from a systems approach, management scientists, lawyers, health scientists, engineers, and other professionals, have great trouble in connecting to the systems idea. The purpose of this book is to fulfill the need for an introduction into systems thinking for the first time student of the subject. It does not pretend to be a comprehensive textbook (the text does assume a reader with an academic background), but to those whose interest has been awakened and who wish to pursue systems thinking, a fairly extensive bibliography is available.

The book is about systems thinking and the application of systems thinking only. There are other texts available that illustrate the benefits of systems practice and its outcomes in real life situations.

Part I is a history of and introduction into systems thinking with the emphasis on human (soft) systems. For the systems student, part II is an example of systems thinking applied to a problem situation in a human activity system.

The book is also intended to contribute towards the debate about health care planning. As such, the intent is not to present a plan or easy solution for the mess in health care. Instead, it is to question some of the assumptions upon which most modern health care planning is based. In other words, it suggests a different way of *thinking* about the problem. In fact, a plan or solution would in many ways be inimical to a systems approach. Most modern approaches to health care planning come from either the hard systems (business management) or social science communities. I believe these approaches to be limited by their inability to plan for complex unstable systems. The systems approach, virtually unknown in the health care sciences, historically developed to deal with precisely such problems. To health care planners therefore, part I serves as an introduction into a philosophy that may be useful for health care planning, and part II, on the basis of this, as a method for rethinking many of the dilemmas that bedevil planning.

The target audience of this book is therefore both students new to systems thinking, as well as health care planners who have not been exposed to systems thinking, not necessarily in that order.

In Part II, systems thinking in general and Churchman's approach in particular are used for an inquiry into health care systems. Medical systems all over the world are on the verge of breakdown, the reason being that neither patients individually, nor governments and business institutions collectively, can afford the delivery of health care as we know it any longer. Due to an increase in knowledge, the concepts of illness processes and the interactions necessary to counteract them have grown from very simple to enormously complex biological and social systems. However, these systems are still approached upon the basis that they can be understood in terms of simple causal chains.

No book can hope to include all possible knowledge available about even a single topic. What I hope to achieve with this book is a bird's eye view, where various aspects of health care are touched upon and synthesized into a new whole. This would not only satisfy the principles of a systems approach, but may also contribute to new ways of thinking about old problems. In the end, all of us are biased by the context of the individual knowledge that serves as the basis that we act upon. Nowhere is this bias more noticeable than in the individual soft systems methodologies. This text is no different. The bias is born out by the application in medicine, but in spite of this, I believe that this book has a contribution to make towards the targeted audiences.

It is customary for the author to thank some of the people who have made a book possible. Firstly and most importantly, I have to thank my wife, Lynne, and my children, Adrian and Tinarie, for stoically bearing my absence during the long hours stolen from them for researching and writing the text. I also have to thank my mentor and friend, Johan Strümpfer, who supported my initiation into systems thinking, and who, during many long discussions tried to impart some of his incredible knowledge and experience of systems to a pupil who had to start a thousand mile journey with a first step away from the ignorance of a professional background. Johann Wessels, friend and artist for the wonderful artwork on the cover to complement the text. Tom Ryan for encouraging me, but more importantly for allowing me access to his department as a systems student. And lastly, but not the least, I would like to thank my parents, who encouraged me from early on to endlessly ask questions about life.

Introduction: Why Should I Use Systems Thinking To Plan?

According to C West Churchman, a manager is the person who makes decisions. Such managers are usually understood to mean professionals with special training, but, in reality, we are all managers. We manage relationships, ourselves, our homes, and so on. Hence, decision-making is an activity that is found at all levels of society. The ability to make proper decisions depends critically on the knowledge we have about a problem situation. The more knowledge we have, and the more accurate the knowledge, the better we can decide. But we also want to be certain that if we act upon the decision we have taken, the outcome will be successful, or that the decision will be executed as planned. In ancient times, people consulted fortune-tellers to predict the future for them (De Geus, 1994). The latter had at their disposal assorted methods to assist them into seeing the future, such as chicken entrails, tarot cards, crystal balls, the stars, bones, and an assortment of miscellaneous items. To our ancestors, nature was unpredictable and mysterious, and forecasting no more than inspired guesswork.

René Descartes is widely considered to be the father of modern philosophy, because he changed the way we think and reason about the ways we search for truth (Hollingdale, 1979; Russell, 1993). His method resulted in the reorganization of science and culminated in the Newtonian system. The way we view the world, even today, is a product of the Cartesian system. According to this view, nature may be likened to a clock or machine (Ackoff, 1981). Machines are regular, predictable, and it is conceptually possible to know everything there is to know about them. Understanding machines requires a method of analysis and reduction, typically described as a three-step approach:

- Divide the problem situation into its smallest components,
- Study the components in order to understand the function and purpose of each, and
- Reassemble them into the whole, upon which knowledge of the function of the whole will result, knowledge that may be used to predict the future successfully.

Machine thinking naturally leads to a belief that all the mysteries and uncertainty of nature may be eradicated by collecting enough knowledge. This, the search for all the knowledge contained in nature is the quest of modern science. Once we believe that we know and understand everything and upon this basis can predict the future, fortune telling becomes obsolete and people who still believe in it are ridiculed for their naiveté and ignorance. In the deterministic world, managers are in control and their orders are executed in response to directives.

In order to make accurate predictions, it is a prerequisite that we shall have accurate knowledge of the initial conditions of the problem state, and also that we shall believe in an environment that shows regularity. These two preconditions are fundamental to the discipline of statistics, a product of machine thinking, of which the purpose is to predict the probability that a certain event or events will take place given selected initial conditions. Statistics, modeling and the belief in a nature that is regular and predictable are basic to modern decision-making and management science.

Machine thinking has been altered somewhat by cybernetic thinking. According to this view, the world is like an organism and requires a brain to manage the other components. The brain thinks for and tells other parts of the organism (system) what to do (Ackoff, 1981). It also interprets the actions of the parts and adjusts further action by new directives, working as a system of control by feedback. In social systems, the brain is represented by management or government, workers are considered not to be purposeful individually, and hence in need of control.

Today, the belief in a mechanismically or organismically conceived world resulted in the replacement of the fortune-teller by the consultant, and astrology, tarot cards and crystal balls by strategic planning, business re-engineering, business analysis and learning organizations. But still, we appear to be only marginally better off. So, what has gone wrong?

There are overwhelming indications that nature consists of an infinite number of components that are linked together in complex webs, rather than being organized as a stable predictable clockwork mechanism (Anderson, 1996). The number of possible permutations for arranging such a system is infinite. Additionally, each component may be influenced by many others in an infinite number of possible ways, thus, an insignificant incident may set into motion a cascade of events that ripple through the system and is only noticed at a point far removed from the original disturbance. This effect is usually illustrated by the proverbial flutter of the wings of a butterfly in Peru that will influence the weather in New York. We are now discovering that complete knowledge of complex systems is impossible. Furthermore, if we plot the increase of knowledge graphically as one axis, and increasing understanding as another, we discover that a point is reached where more knowledge results in less understanding as a result of information overload. In complex systems, some regularity can be discovered scientifically, but many interactions are the result of one of many possible future states that result in unique new features, the path of which cannot be predicted in advance.

Heisenberg's Law confirms what we have come to suspect, in unpredictable systems initial conditions cannot be known with certainty and future states can therefore not be predicted with any sort of accuracy at all. In short, questions are being asked about the validity of current belief systems and the source and accuracy of our knowledge (Kvale, 1996).

Planning and management does not escape the results of uncertainty either. Most plans are either not implemented at all, or in a manner different from what was intended (Stacey, 1992). The cause is the difficulty in knowing initial conditions, difficulty in predicting outcomes of interventions accurately, and a world that is not stable and regular.

Sometimes, plans are spectacularly successful, but we wished it had not been, because success also opens Pandora's box and allows out demons that are often worse than the original problem (Vickers, 1980). The thunder of elephant feet in complex systems creates more havoc than the flutter of butterfly wings. Through science, we have learnt to use and harness the forces of nature, but not how to control it. The cause is machine thinking. In reality, what we observe as stability or regularity in nature, is the result of internal self-regulation effected by the way that components interact. If we nudge a system, the ripple effect set into motion often destabilizes that which ensures regularity in the first place The notion of control by a brain in complex systems therefore has no meaning. We must be aware that social systems are no different in this respect from other complex systems.

If the belief in machine or organismic systems is no longer tenable, one may be tempted to nihilism and the avoidance of decision-making altogether in the absence of an alternative (Kvale, 1996). People are naturally averse to risk taking in decision-making, which makes perfect sense. I would rather make a successful decision that will lead to promotion and an increase in salary, than an adverse one that my result in my dismissal (De Geus, 1994). The alternative would be to construct an approach complementary to the facts of nature, as we understand them today.

The features of such an approach would have to include the following:

- Even if we cannot know everything about nature, we can attempt to understand the complexity of problem situations in terms of the complex whole.
- With such understanding, we may gain insight into the interactions behind what we observe as regularity and consequently the effects on the containing whole of changes we make.

- Knowledge of the complexity of nature and what regulates it requires a system of thinking at a metalevel that may lead to an understanding of wholes.
- We cannot achieve the ideal of complete knowledge of nature or even a problem situation, but we can attempt to overcome this deficiency through knowledge of the history of the problem, and by understanding as many perspectives about it as possible.
- It is possible to commit oneself to an ideal, defined as a goal we cannot achieve, but that we can approach indefinitely. Ongoing progress requires a commitment to making perpetual adjustments towards the ideal in response to unforeseen changes in the environment.
- Complex systems are internally controlled by self-regulation and it is possible to make adjustments to what regulates the system.
- Social systems represent some of the most complex interactions known to us. Control in such systems is impossible, apart from by coercion. But it is possible to solicit the co-operation of individuals and to achieve in this way aligned self-control. Such an approach requires a belief in humans as purposeful entities in their own right and therefore the acceptance of a social system metaphor of human activity.

In short, we need to rediscover the ancient wisdom of the interconnectedness of nature as a whole. We may benefit, if we make alterations to systems to improve the working of the whole, without causing new unwanted effects. On this road of discovery, we need guides, not gurus.

This description of an approach to planning more closely aligned with present day knowledge of the life that surrounds us, in effect describes a systems approach. The systems approach is neither crystal bowl nor recipe. Instead, it is a system of wisdom to change what we can, leave alone what we cannot or should not, and the ability to tell the difference.

No doubt, the astute reader would have detected in this section the description of postmodernity and the dilemmas associated with it[1]. It is likely that post-modern science will be transformed based upon the notions of

---

[1] The term "postmodern" can be understood as no longer living in the "modern" world, and "modern" as the time of the Enlightenment, lasting roughly from the eighteenth until the twentieth century (Anderson, 1996). In effect, what we are experiencing today is the breakdown of the "Enlightenment project".

wholism, interconnection, and self-regulation (Appignanesi and Garratt, 1995). As we have argued, systems thinking is the one discipline handily placed to lead in this transformation, or paradigm shift.

Part 1: Systems Thinking

Chapter 1: An Archaeology Of Systems And Related Thinking

Understanding the systems idea requires an understanding of the history of Western philosophy. René Descartes (1596 - 1650), the father of modern philosophy (Hollingdale, 1966) was the first philosopher since Aristotle to attempt a reconstruction of philosophy and the first thinker whose outlook was influenced by the new paradigms in physics and astronomy (Russell, 1961). His system also served as the basis for the later rationalist school of thinking.

Rationalism is the theory that knowledge of the actual world can be attained by a process of reason divorced from personal experience (Hollingdale, 1966). Apart from Descartes, the great rationalist philosophers were Benedict de Spinoza (1632 - 1677) and Wilhelm Leibniz (1646 - 1716). From these names, it can be seen that rationalism had its greatest influence on the continent of Europe. A group of English philosophers, starting with Francis Bacon (1561 - 1626), and more importantly, continued by John Locke (1632 - 1704), later George Berkeley (1685 - 1753), and David Hume (1711 - 1776) reacted to rationalism with the opposing theory that all knowledge of the actual word derives from personal experience, a position known as *empiricism*.

Immanuel Kant (1724 - 1804) attempted to reconcile rationalism and empiricism in a school that became known as *transcendental idealism*. He studied in the Leibnizian school of philosophy, but later rejected its laws in favor of a position that included aspects of Rousseau's romanticism and Hume's empiricism. George Hegel's (1770 - 1831) philosophy revived rationalism, causing a second English reaction, culminating in *positivism*, or modern empiricism. Most modern schools of thought, of whom the most important is logical positivism, are considered to be extensions of empiricism. Logical positivism is known in particular for the Vienna circle: Moritz Schlick (1882 - 1936), Rudolf Carnap (1891 - 1970), Kurt Gödel (1906 - 1978), and others, who were influenced in their thinking by the traditional empiricists, but also by Bertrand Russell (1872 - 1970), Ludwig Wittgenstein (1889 - 1951), and others. Modern rationalism is represented mainly in metaphysics, theology and ethics. Schopenhauer (1788 - 1860) explored the more metaphysical aspects of Kant's system into a tradition that was continued by Friedrich Nietzsche (1844 - 1900), who in turn had an appreciable influence on Jean-Paul Sartre (1905 - 1980) and other existentialist thinkers.

Karl Marx (1818 - 1883) although having influenced social thinking in a profound way, is considered by many writers in philosophy not to be a philosopher by definition. He studied Hegelian philosophy and developed a system of thought called *dialectic materialism*, based upon Hegel's more radical ideas. The Frankfurt school of sociology: Theodor Adorno (1903 - 1969), Max Horkheimer (1895 - 1973), Herbert Marcuse (1898 - 1979), and others, continued the Marxist tradition with their *critical theory*, of which the most modern exponent is Jürgen Habermas (born 1929).

From a systems point view the founding of the school of *pragmatism*[1] in America is important. Credit for this theory is given to CS Peirce (1839 - 1914) (Hookway, 1985), although William James (1842 - 1910) later employed the term pragmatism to mean something different. Peirce graduated in chemistry, but later lectured in philosophy. He was influenced by reading Kant and Schiller, which stimulated an interest in forming an understanding of the underpinnings of logic and particularly meaning as a foundation for logic. He wanted to prove that correct inquiry would lead to knowledge of an objective reality. James, a psychologist, on the other hand, understood pragmatism to mean that truth is what is good from a human point of view, or, truth is an idea made true by events. The other major influence on the school of pragmatism is John Dewey (1859 - 1910). We shall see later that Edgar Singer was a student of James and C West Churchman, an important contributor to the systems idea, in turn a student of Singer. Hence, pragmatism and by extension Kantian idealism is fundamental to the systems philosophy.

Science as we knew it at the beginning of the twentieth century was not only a product of Western civilization, but also a relic of the Cartesian system. Scientists believed that the fundamental laws of the universe are deterministic and reversible (Checkland, 1991). Hence, processes that occurred outside these laws were taken to be artifacts, exceptions, or due to a lack of sufficient knowledge. New laws were researched within the laboratory and it was assumed that the researcher is an observer and decision-maker apart from the systems under observation. Furthermore, it was assumed that the system under observation itself is under control of deterministic laws and that to study them, conditions in the laboratory could be closed to influences from the environment. Today we know that in the study of the universal laws of science in general and human sciences in particular, we are both observers and participants at the same time. Furthermore, it is now becoming clear that our world is not stable and predictable, but unstable. In unstable systems, small changes in initial

---

[1] Also called instrumentalism

conditions may lead to large amplifications of effects in time that has a negative effect on predictability.

New paradigms became necessary to explain the complex self-organizing systems that traditional science failed to explain, since such systems represent a significant part of what we experience as life. One such theory that has been gaining ground rapidly is systems thinking. The reason for this is that the systems approach is a *meta*-approach that transcends many disciplines and philosophies. Hence, a major advantage is that it provides a way for approaching complex real world problems that defy the usual deterministic approaches. Secondly, it provides a way for understanding how the environment works without having to study each of its parts in great detail (Kauffman, 1980).

According to Appignanesi and Garratt (1995), a post-modern revolution in science is likely, based upon the notions of holism, interconnection, and autonomous self-governance. These notions are fundamental to the systems idea and it would be fair to say that the systems approach has the potential to become an important modern scientific paradigm.

General Systems Theory

It is widely acknowledged that Ludwig Von Bertalanffy, a biologist, was the first to articulate the concepts that are accepted today as the foundations of a *general systems theory* (GST) (Checkland, 1991; Von Bertalanffy, 1968)[2]. He first published these ideas in 1947 and incorporated philosophical concepts, which, according to him, were influenced by the work of Leibniz, Paracelsus, Hegel, and the more recent gestalt theory of Wolfgang Köhler (1887 - 1967), and also by his association with Moritz Schlick and Hans Reichenbach (1891 - 1953) (of the Vienna Circle), Herzberg (a psychologist), and Parsefal (an engineer). Together with Anatol Rapoport (a biomathematician), Kenneth Boulding (1910 - 1993)(an economist), and Ralph Gerard (a physiologist), Von Bertalanffy founded the *Society for General Systems Research* (SGSR) in 1954. The origins of the systems approach therefore reflect its aim of being a meta-discipline. The name of the Society was later changed to the *International Society for General Systems Research* (ISGSR) and is known today as the *International Society for Systems Science* (ISSS).

---

[2]According to Sadovsky and Kelle, there are reasons to believe that Von Bertalanffy may have been influenced by reading Alexander Bogdanov's (a pseudonym used by Alexander Malinovsky (1873 - 1928)) book, Tektology (Dudley, 1996), since the idea of tektology bears a remarkable similarity in many ways to GST. The point is moot, since Von Bertalanffy spread the gospel, so to speak, and therefore may rightfully lay claim to being the founder of the systems movement. Besides, many texts, even as far back as that of the Greek philosophers, contain ideas that probably predate the final synthesis of systems thinking.

Cybernetics[3,4]

Norbert Wiener's *cybernetics*, Shannon and Weaver's *information theory*, and Von Neumann and Morgenstern's *game theory* developed in parallel to and influenced systems thinking. Wiener's work was of particular importance, since it introduced the concepts of feedback, self-regulation, and the flow of information in complex systems. These are important considerations, as will be shown later, for determining multiple complex relations, for the exchange of information in systems, and as a foundation for control theory. Wiener (1894 - 1964), Von Neumann (1903 - 1957), Shannon (born 1916) and Weaver (1894 - 1978) were all mathematicians, and hence were searching for empirical solutions to communication and information processing. This is understandable, since modern positivism has an interest in semantics and the use of language.

General Living Systems Theory

Alfred North Whitehead (1861 - 1947), mathematician and philosopher, conceived an approach to the problems of science similar to that of general systems theory at about the same time that Von Bertalanffy published the results of his work. He called his approach the *philosophy of organism* (Miller, 1978). Life, according to him, was made up of a system of systems, similar in many respects to the way that organisms are organized. A student of his, James Grier Miller, expanded this philosophy into *living systems theory* (LST), which has a significant following. Related conceptually to LST is Jaros and Cloete's *biomatrix theory* (Tracy, 1995).

According to Miller, all living systems consist of a hierarchy of seven levels. In addition, each of these levels is subdivided into another nineteen critical subsystems that are essential for supporting life (Miller, 1978). Purposeful behavior is considered to be fundamental to all living systems, and the aim of behavior is to achieve a steady state (Tracy, 1995). Purpose is considered to be an internal steady state, goals preferred external states, or relationships, and learning may modify both.

Biomatrix theory views living systems as composed of self-governing subsystems called teleons, which in turn may by purpose-directed (endoteleons) or goal directed (exoteleons). Both LST and biomatrix theory

---

[3] The term *cybernetics* is derived from the Greek word steersman (Churchman, 1968). To stay on course to a destination, the steersman of the boat has to continuously adjust the direction of travel in response to signals indicating that the direction of travel is off target.

[4] According to Bateson (1979), cybernetics may be defined as: a branch of mathematics dealing with problems of control, recursiveness, and information.

conceives systems as organismic and strictly hierarchical and is substantially influenced by cybernetic principles, which reflect their origin in the biological sciences.

Hard Systems

During the Second World War, scientifically trained civilians were used to assist in the planning of military operations (Ackoff, 1981; Checkland, 1991; Churchman, 1968a; Churchman, 1979). After the war, the RAND[5] Corporation continued using the experience gained by them and it also formed the basis of the new discipline of *operational research*[6] (OR). The RAND approach (also known as *systems analysis*) was eventually systematized into the economic appraisal of:

- Various alternative means available for attaining defined ends; and
- The costs and consequences for attaining them.

The RAND methodology is fundamental to most modern business management approaches and may be summarized as follows.

- There is a desired state S_1 and a present state S_0.
- There are alternative ways for getting from S_0 to S_1.
- The problem is solved by defining S_1 and S_0 and by selecting the best means for reducing the difference between them.

Operational Research on the other hand, is often used for the scientific control of human and mechanical systems (Ackoff, quoted in Von Bertalanffy, 1968). Systems thinking is also basic to *systems engineering* (SE) (also known as engineering management), which developed separately from, and in parallel to the RAND approach and OR as a subdiscipline of traditional engineering. SE may be defined as the task of conceiving, designing, evaluating, and implementing a system to meet some defined need (Checkland, 1991). This definition fulfils the technological goal of engineering namely the most efficient accomplishment of a defined end.

The belief that problems may be formulated in the ways described above is fundamental to all hard systems. Philosophically, they are empirical, and scientifically orientated, and therefore concerned with model building, statistics, and mathematics - formulation being important to their methodologies. Such approaches work well for complex structured problems with clear goals, but it rapidly became apparent that they are less successful

---

[5]An acronym for research and development
[6]Known as *operational* research in the UK and *operations* research in the USA (Churchman, 1979).

when dealing with unstructured problems with poorly defined boundaries and ends. Such problems are common to human activity systems and approaches designed specifically to deal with them are called soft systems approaches.[7] Human activity systems will be the focus of interest for the rest of the text.

Soft Systems

No individual can claim the credit for being the founder of the soft systems stream of systems thinking. However, the contribution of C West Churchman (born 1913) stands out by virtue of the scope and depth of his work (Ulrich, 1988). Churchman studied philosophy under Edgar A Singer, who in turn was a student of William James, well known for his contribution to philosophical pragmatism. Singer insisted on comprehensiveness when inquiring into the natural world (Churchman, 1979). This means that scientific inquiry cannot exclude values from decision-making. Furthermore, to add to knowledge, the scope of inquiry has to be widened (more information should be swept in), rather than narrowed down in a traditional approach of reduction.

After World War II, Churchman became a pioneering member of operational research and is the author of the first textbook in this discipline (Ulrich, 1988). However, he felt constrained by the rigidity of the methodology of OR and his belief in comprehensiveness lead him to the systems approach, an approach that blended more naturally with his thinking and in which he published widely. Many soft systems methodologies have his writings as their basis, including interactive planning (Russell Ackoff was his first PhD student), critical systems heuristics (Werner Ulrich was another student of his), strategic assumption surfacing and testing, and soft systems methodology (Richard Mason, Ian Mitroff, and Peter Checkland were all influenced by their association with Churchman). Churchman's work is considered to be of fundamental importance as a systems philosophy, and will be summarized in a later chapter.

In the 1970's, another major contribution to soft systems thinking was made when Peter Checkland, a systems engineer, influenced by his experience of the inability of systems engineering to deal effectively with ill-structured complex problems, actively started researching ways for solving them. The experience was formalized as *soft systems methodology* (SSM). He arrived at a methodology not dissimilar to Churchman's, and Ulrich's critical systems heuristics (CSH), but from a different philosophical basis. Checkland used

---

[7]The terms hard and soft systems were coined by Peter Checkland (1991)

concepts of action research (based upon Kurt Lewin's field theory[8]) to arrive at a methodology that works in practice.

Checkland believes that problems arise when people have contrasting perceptions of the same situation. Intervention is therefore effected by:

- A process of inquiry that leads to purposeful action in a continuous cycle (a learning system).
- The recognition of cultural constraints (in the broadest sense).
- Participation in planning by all those involved in the system.
- Thinking about the problem using systems thinking on the one hand and real world thinking on the other (a dialectic).

SSM is a powerful methodology that is useful for dealing with problems in which consensus is possible. The problem though, with a theory that is derived entirely upon practical experience, is that it has a problem to establish the reasons for its success, and Checkland succumbed to the temptation to retrospectively establish a philosophical basis for SSM (Checkland, 1981). According to him, SSM is a learning system that may be embedded within phenomenology, hermeneutics and critical theory.

Systems methodologies

Today, there are six (soft) systems methodologies used individually or in combination to solve complex problems in human activity systems. These are:

　i. System dynamics (SD)
　ii. Viable system diagnosis (VSD)
　iii. Strategic assumption surfacing and testing (SAST)
　iv. Interactive planning (IP)
　v. Soft systems methodology (SSM)
　vi. Critical systems heuristics (CSH)

System dynamics (originally known as industrial dynamics) is the result of the work of Jay Forrester at the Massachusetts Institute of Technology (MIT). Forrester's interest changed from Electro-mechanical research to the application of feedback control to socio-economic systems. SD is a theory of information feedback and control, and therefore applies cybernetic concepts to complex systems. Control engineers use similar concepts in linear and non-linear control theory. It is a useful method for determining the structure of, and processes in systems under study, but SD, although contributing significantly towards an understanding of complex causal relations, cannot

---

[8]Lewin (1890 - 1947) was a psychologist of the gestalt school

deal with those factors that are central to the function and regulation of complex human interactions. The reason is that SD modeling is based upon an expression of simultaneous non-linear integral differential equations, a form of mathematics, hence the SD tradition is empirical and mechanismic.

Systems thinking, as SD, is part of Peter Senge's *learning organization* approach, which is popular in some sections of management science. Senge's approach consists of five components (Senge, 1990):

   i. Systems thinking.
   ii. Personal mastery.
   iii. Mental models.
   iv. Building a shared vision.
   v. Team learning.

Systems thinking is conceptualized as a tool for making complex patterns clearer. Managers, are meant to use this approach to test the mental models upon which perceptions in organizations are based, in addition driven by a wish for personal growth. Aligning mental models assist in building shared visions, group learning and therefore more efficient organization. The underlying metaphor is organismic.

Viable system diagnosis, in common with SD, focuses on the complex interactions taking place within organizations. It is the product of an expansion of cybernetic principles by Stafford Beer. The focus is on organization and control, and in common with all cybernetically conceived models, the operative metaphor is organismic. This approach has the same shortcomings as SD, both being more suitable for dealing with simple unitary problems.

Strategic assumption surfacing and testing[9] focuses on the relationship between the participants in a problem context. Their differences are debated and underlying assumptions about the problem brought to the fore. In this way, consensus may be achieved, and it is assumed that remaining problems may then be resolved by ordinary management techniques. The methodology owes its philosophical basis to Churchman, and Kantian apriori and Hegelian consensus in particular, figure prominently. SAST is useful for dealing with relatively simple problems where there is a compatibility of interest and compromise is possible.

---

[9]SAST is the creation of Richard Mason and Ian Mitroff. Mitroff later worked with Harold Linstone, originator of the multiple perspectives approach (MPA), related conceptually to SAST, and a very useful methodology for bringing out multiple perspectives in a problem situation (Mitroff and Linstone, 1993; Linstone and Mitroff, 1994).

Russell Ackoff's career started off with an undergraduate degree in architecture, and a PhD in philosophy under Churchman. His *interactive planning* is based upon the idea that decision makers ought to assist those that participate in an organization, to design a desirable future for themselves. It assumes as fundamental that planning ought to be continuous, holistic, and participative, and that design ought to be based upon an ideal that may not be achieved for a long time, but may be approached indefinitely. In order to adapt to a rapidly changing environment, a process of learning by members of the organization is required. The contribution of Churchman and the pragmatic tradition to this philosophy is significant, and none more so than the insistence on the inclusion of values in design. The operative metaphor in IP is the social system metaphor (which will be discussed later), hence this approach has particular relevance for dealing with the problems of human activity systems.

The methodology that is probably the closest philosophically and conceptually to Churchman's systems theory is Werner Ulrich's *critical systems heuristics*. Ulrich studied business administration and economy, and holds a PhD in social systems design, for which he also studied under Churchman. CSH is particularly strong for critically reflecting upon the consensus achieved, and changes brought about by planning. Ulrich distinguishes between the mechanismic and organismic thinking of what he calls systems science (OR, systems analysis, SE, SD, and cybernetics), dominated by how things *should* be done, on the one hand, and critical systems thinking on the other, that is concerned with what *ought* to be done. This implies a freedom of choice to design and improve human systems, and a concern for those who have to live the consequences of planning. The strength of CSH is in dealing with problems that inherently contain a high level of coercion. CSH is philosophically deeply indebted to Kantian dialectic, Churchman's systems theory, and Jürgen Habermas' critical theory.

No discussion of soft systems would be complete without mentioning Michael Jackson and Bob Flood's *critical systems thinking* (CST). Traditional management science came under attack for accepting existing structures of inequality in society, and by doing so, perpetuating them (Jackson, 1991). In a search for alternatives, these authors turned to systems thinking. Critical Systems Thinking is based upon five commitments:

  i. Critical awareness.
 ii. Social awareness.
iii. Complementarism at the methodological level.
 iv. Complementarism at the theoretical level; and
  v. Dedication to human emancipation.

Considering these commitments, an attempt is made to understand the strengths and weaknesses of the theoretical underpinnings of the available systems methodologies. This may lead to an awareness of the possible consequences when any of these methodologies are applied. Furthermore, such an understanding is useful for identifying those circumstances where each methodology will be maximally effective. Based upon a critique of soft systems thinking, Jackson arrived at a system of systems methodologies, which he and Flood refined into what they consider to be a meta-methodology called *total systems intervention* (TSI) (Flood and Jackson, 1991). The philosophical basis of CST is Habermas' critical theory, a modification of the neo-Marxist Frankfurt School's social philosophy, and is aimed at achieving human emancipation.

Upon reflection, one may conclude that Churchman's systems theory, an extension of pragmatism and therefore practical philosophy, forms the backbone of soft systems thinking. Some of the systems methodologies lack the underpinning of well-developed theory, which impacts on their applicability. This problem plays out the traditional dialectic between science and technology; the one focused on theory and not practice, and the other on practice and not theory. On the one hand, systems thinking needs to show that it has practical application in real life, but on the other, there is a danger in it being seen as merely a tool by managers, without them understanding the importance of its philosophical background.

Studies Of Complexity, Chaos And Non-Linearity

The last, and most recent, historical strand associated with holistic thinking, is that of the studies of *complexity* and *non-linear systems*, which became more mainstream in the 1960's as a result of the work of Edward Lorenz, a meteorologist (Gleick, 1987). Scientists from many diverse disciplines participated in founding the Santa Fe Institute in the 1980's, since then associated with the studies of complexity. The approach is mainly an attempt to find logical patterns in complex processes, definable in mathematical terms. Complex systems in general have some features in common (Waldrop, 1992):

- Complex systems tend to undergo spontaneous self-organization.
- Complex systems actively adapt to changing environments and therefore constantly evolve.
- Complex systems often stabilize on the edge between order and chaos (edge of chaos), where they are stable enough to be self sustaining, and where the environment is disordered enough to ensure sufficient variety so that stagnation will not occur.

There are studies that show that large complex systems self-organize to a critical state in which even minor events may initiate reactions of catastrophic proportions (Bak and Kan, 1991). This is typical of chaotic systems, characterized by random behavior that may be generated by orderly non-linear systems (Crutchfield et al. 1986; Kauffman, 1991). In such systems, initial conditions that are very much alike may have markedly different outcomes, since small uncertainties are amplified disproportionately (in a non-linear fashion) as a result of which long-term predictions are impossible. Complex systems tend to self-organize around *attractors* that are selected at random (antichaos).

It is noteworthy that in the past, based upon Cannon's concept of homeostasis, it was assumed that physiological systems seek stability. Studies based upon the concepts of non-linearity and chaos have shown the opposite to be true. Healthy systems are irregular, and regularity may be an indication of pathology, because of an inability to respond to challenges from the environment (Goldberger et al. 1990). Of further interest is that many parts of living systems show *fractal*[10] patterns, which may shed light on some aspects of their development. Examples are the vascular and bronchial trees.

Although the studies into the physical nature of complex systems are not considered part of systems thinking at present, they, and particularly studies of artificial life systems, may in time contribute to a better understanding of complex systems, particularly living systems.

Unfortunately, the term "system" is often used in a number of contexts, related and unrelated to the systems approach, and is therefore a source of confusion. One such unrelated context is computer systems, studied by systems analysts. It is my belief that the term "wholism" would be an appropriate substitute for systems of the kind discussed in this book. However, for the moment, we have to stay in the mainstream and refer to systems thinking and the systems approach, rather than wholismic thinking and the wholismic approach.

At this point, the reader should have a clearer idea of where the systems approach originated from, and how it is related contextually to the other disciplines with which it is often confused. Also, in this chapter we saw the historical development of general systems theory as a philosophy and its eventual practical application as hard and soft systems approaches. In the

---

[10]A *fractal* is an object that reveals more detail of a self-similar nature as it is increasingly magnified (Goldberger et al. 1990).

next chapter, we shall take a closer look at some of the fundamentals of systems thinking.

Chapter 2: Systems Concepts

In the real world, we constantly have to deal with complex phenomena. They are complex because they have no easy rational explanations and are the source of problem situations that are usually difficult to describe, often recognizable only as unease. When the discomfort <u>can</u> be described, it may not be possible to accurately define or circumscribe the extent of the situation. The ability to deal with such "wicked" problems depends critically upon the knowledge we have about the situation, and a large part of our behavior therefore is characterized by inquiry, or the search for proper knowledge before we act. Business planning, research, and medical diagnosis are examples of every day inquiry (Strümpfer, 1992).

Diagram 1: A Hierarchy of Knowledge

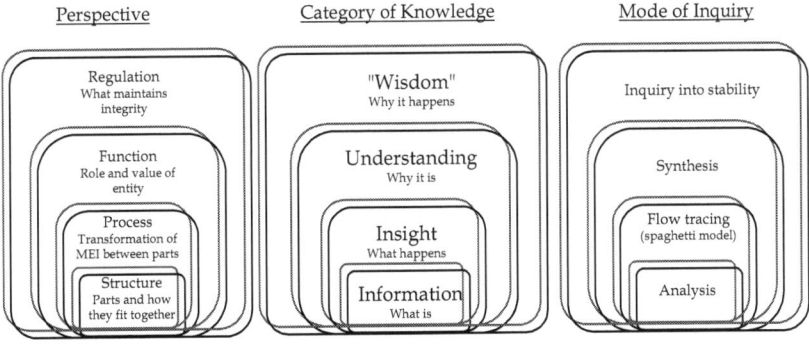

(Adapted from Strümpfer (1994) with permission from the author)

The systems approach is a powerful method for gaining useful knowledge of the kind necessary for decision-making that can be rationally defended. A systems based system of knowledge can be categorized into the following hierarchy; information, insight, understanding, and wisdom. As illustrated in **diagram 1**, each level of knowledge is included in the next (higher) level, with wisdom being the highest, and hence the most complete form of knowledge upon which a decision may be made.

Information is knowledge about how things fit together statically, and therefore refers to stability and equilibrium (i.e. *structure*, or *what is*). Insight is knowledge about the dynamics of a system, and therefore refers to the flow and transformation of MEI[1] (i.e. *process, or what happens*). Understanding is knowledge about a system's external relations, and therefore refers to *function* and purpose, or *why it is*. Lastly, "wisdom"[2] is knowledge about what keeps components together, and therefore refers to regulation and *stability, or why things happen*.

The legacy of the Cartesian system to scientific method is *analysis*, a three-step process traditionally applied as follows (Ackoff, 1981).

   i.   Reduce the thing to be understood to its parts.
   ii. Try to understand the behavior of each part.
   iii. Then try to understand the whole by reassembling the parts.

Take for example attempts to understand the functioning of the human body. Analysis starts by dissecting the body into its parts (gross anatomy). The parts can be divided into cells and cellular components by respectively microscopy, and electron microscopy (histology). The cellular components and processes are in turn reduced in terms of biochemical processes (physiology), and biochemistry, in turn, depends on an understanding of physics. All the components are traditionally reassembled into the practice of medicine.

The purpose of analysis is to explain *how* things work and the product of analysis is *knowledge*. All modern scientific and technological (hard system) thinking is of the analytic kind. The problem is that in real terms, knowledge of parts does *not* translate into an understanding of wholes. Hence, wholismic thinking requires a process with features that are the exact opposite to analysis, namely *synthesis*.

   i.   Identify the *whole* of which the thing to be explained of is part.
   ii. Explain the behavior and properties of the *whole*.
   iii. Then explain the behavior and properties of the thing to be explained in terms of its *relationship* to the whole.

Synthesis explains *why* things work as they do (function) and therefore results in *understanding*. It is important to understand that analytic and synthetic thinking is not mutually exclusive, but complementary, and that in systems thinking they are used as such.

---

[1] Matter, energy and information.
[2] Strümpfer uses the term "wisdom" in inverted commas to differentiate it from the much wider common meaning as is usually understood.

The purpose of the rest of the chapter is to introduce the reader to the fundamentals of wholismic (systems) thinking. We shall see that a system consists of parts that stand together to form a whole. Understanding of the whole may be gained in terms of the *structure* and *process* of the system. Components of systems may combine to form higher hierarchical levels, with each new level showing properties that are unique to that level (*emergence*). The parts partake in process by the exchange of information that in turn is used to regulate the system by a process of feedback. In this way the system is stabilized, but the price for stability is the constraints that are necessary to control.

Living systems are open to the environment and perfect equilibrium is therefore not possible. In addition, to maintain the structure of living systems, all of its components have to co-operate. This requires a constant exchange of information between individual components so that they may adjust, the direction of which must be transmitted to other components so that they may adjust as well in the same direction, and so on. In other words, constant self-regulation of the components takes place in response to a constant exchange of information with the environment. The components therefore respond not only to information about other components, but also to information about the system's environment.

An important feature of living systems is that they respond *purposefully* to new signals.

Definition of a system

The word *system* is derived from the Greek verb *sunistánai*, which means to cause to stand together (Bowler, 1981; Flood and Jackson, 1991; Patching, 1990; Senge, 1994; Von Bertalanffy, 1968). In other words, systems are made up of sets of interconnected components that act together to function as a whole. In a system, components display properties that are properties of the whole, rather than properties of the components (Checkland, 1991; Churchman, 1968a; Kauffman, 1980). Hence, according to Ackoff (1981)(see also Strümpfer, 1994b), in a system:

- The behavior of each component has an effect on the behavior of the whole.
- The behavior of components and their effects on the whole are interdependent; and
- There are no components without an effect on the behavior of the whole, and the effect depends on the effect on other components.

It follows that a system (as a whole) cannot be divided into independent components; each component has properties that are lost if the component is separated from the whole, and the system as a whole has properties that none of the parts has (Ackoff, 1981).

For example, each part of the human body has an effect on the whole body. A properly functioning respiratory system ensures the proper functioning of the brain, muscles, and so on; the brain ensures the proper functioning of the lungs, heart, muscles, and so on and so forth. This example stresses the fact that the effect of each organ on the body depends on at least one other organ; the effect of the respiratory system, for example, depends mostly on the effect of the vascular system. Lastly, none of the organs can be combined into a purposeful system apart from the body, since they lose their function when separated from the whole.

Diagram 2: System Viewpoints

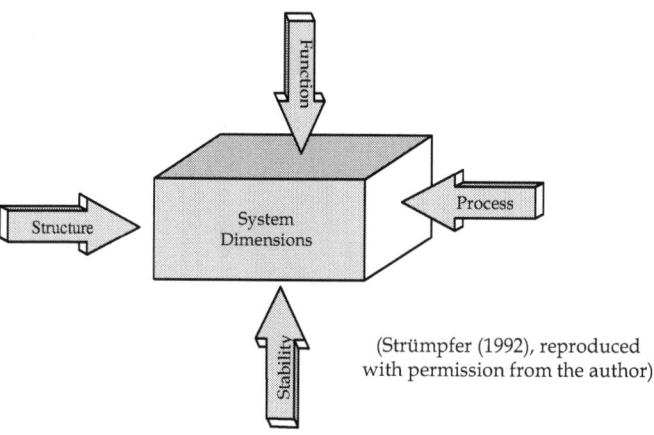

(Strümpfer (1992), reproduced with permission from the author)

Possibly the greatest contribution of systems thinking to rational decision-making is its ability to direct the inquirer to look at a problematic system from many perspectives - one may liken this to looking at a cube (see **diagram 2**). This, the ability to include multiple perspectives in the process of understanding is, a profound insight and fundamental to systems thinking.

As described before, there are four major perspectives from which a system may be viewed, namely:

i. Structure
ii. Process
iii. Function
iv. Regulation

Structure

Structure refers to the pattern of interrelationships amongst the components of the system that remain relatively stable (unchanged) over the period of time that the system is under investigation (Bowler, 1981; Senge, 1994).

All complex systems are constructed out of interconnected components (subsystems) that form a *hierarchy*[3], or levels of organization, each more complex than the foregoing. A higher level of organization is recognized by *emergent properties*, or the novel relationships that are properties unique to that level of organization, but meaningless to the level below (Checkland, 1991). Individual components cannot exhibit these properties and they are lost when the system dissolves. For example, the relationship between muscles, bones, brain and other organs makes it possible to play the piano. The ability to be a piano playing system is lost if any of these organs are lost or malfunctioning. It is important to realize that a hierarchy of systems is a continuum from the "simplest" atomic system to the most complex living system. Many authors have attempted to design a taxonomy of systems in order to demonstrate a hierarchy of systems (see for example Bowler (1981) and Miller (1978)), but boundaries between systems in the end are artificial and unstable and, although useful for studying systems, often represent only a snapshot of a system in time. Ultimately, the decision to separate a system from the whole is an arbitrary one for the purpose of study and in no way should be confused with reality.

Once an entity of interest has been identified as part of a system, analytic thinking may be applied for gaining information about the components making up the system and the ways that they are structurally related. This results in knowledge about the system under observation.

Process

Process refers to the relationships that change during the period of investigation. The term embraces both ongoing functions (the flow of matter/energy/information through, and its transformation by the system)(see **diagram 3**), as well as the past history of the system (Miller, 1978).

---

[3]*Hierarchy* may be defined as a set of relations in which units are organised into more inclusive wholes (Bowler, 1981).

Diagram 3: The Transformation of MEI

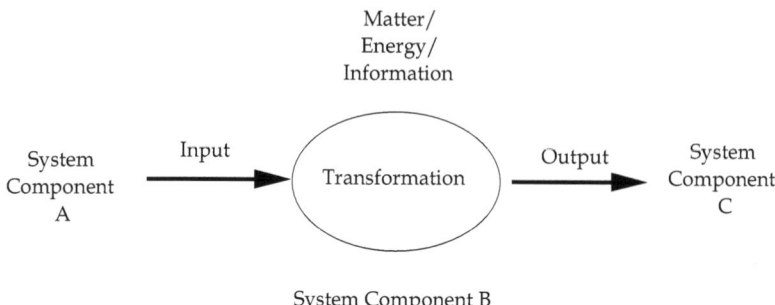

Rudolf Clausius recognized the importance of a system's disorder (*entropy*[4]), as a measure of its efficiency in converting MEI (De Vree, 1994). The amount of MEI in closed systems is constant (first law of thermodynamics). Energy can be transformed from one form into another, but cannot be created or destroyed. Matter, energy and information are closely related[5], and in material systems containing energy, matter has to be transformed to set the energy free, a process in turn dependant on using energy set free by the decay of other systems. The amount of energy available to perform work is related to the degree of organization (*negentropy*) of the matter, or, in other words, the creation of order requires work. If energy is unavailable for work, the most probable state of the system is disordered equilibrium (entropy) (second law of thermodynamics). On the other hand, to *maintain* a stable ordered state, requires a constant input of energy. Ordered systems are more predictable than disordered systems, because the components of the latter have a larger number of possible states available to select from, which negatively impacts on prediction.

The relationships between individual subsystems, and between subsystems and the system as a whole, are often in opposition (*polarity*), and therefore a source of tension. In order to protect the integrity of the system, the system constantly seeks to overcome this tension by attempting to balance the polar

---

[4]*Entropy* is the degree to which the relations between components of any system are mixed up, unsorted, undifferentiated, and random (Bateson, 1979).
[5]$E=mc^2$.

opposites. This balancing process requires a constant input of information about the present state of a system, and a standard against which the information can be compared. If there is a discrepancy, the system is adjusted in order to remain between the boundaries determined by the standard.

Equilibrium, or balance, is possible in systems closed to the environment[6], but open systems constantly exchange information (communicate) with their environments and respond to the information received. Hence, such systems continuously adapt (change) in response to new signals and equilibrium is not possible. The process by which the system seeks to attain equilibrium in open systems is called *equilibration*. Most open systems are able to attain a stable state when the processes that they are involved in are regulated between confined boundaries. This state is often referred to as *equifinality*.

When components become part of a system, they not only become related to the system, but also constrained by their relations within the system. All entities are parts of some systems, even though this may not be obvious at first. Hence, being part of the system discriminates against some of the variety of possibilities that may otherwise be available to the subsystem.[7] In other words, the component gives up some of the possible choices available to it, in return for the benefits that accrue from being part of the system as a whole. If constraints break down, the components of the system are free to seek new relationships or patterns of behavior (Bowler, 1981). In social systems, participation is a matter of choice, but by becoming part of a system, the constraints of participation have to be accepted. In return, individuals benefit from those functions of the system that would be unavailable to them as individual entities functioning on their own. For example, joining a library is a matter of choice, but by doing so, the individual must agree to subscribe to the rules of the system, such as returning books on time, and so on. Individuals may have separate book collections, but none are able to put together a collection as large or comprehensive as that of a library, hence, by accepting the regulations, a larger body of knowledge becomes available to them.

To generate insight about a system, knowledge about the flow of MEI through the system, in other words about process, is necessary. System dynamics modeling and an understanding of multiple complex causality are both useful, and a requirement, for insight. Complex causality will be discussed later in the text.

---

[6]Conventional physics deals with closed systems (Von Bertalanffy, 1968).
[7]A *relation* is a connection between two or more systems that operates as a constraint on the behaviour of the system as a whole (Bowler, 1981).

Function

Function refers to the novel or new relationships that become possible because of the system's stable internal relationships (Strümpfer, 1992). These are the emergent properties referred to earlier, in other words, it refers to a system's role, value, or purpose to another bigger system. For example, health care as a system only has meaning relative to the function it fulfills as component of the larger social system to which it belongs. Note that function refers to the specific relationship between an entity and a particular context.

In medicine, anatomy is the discipline that studies the structure of the human body, and physiology the one associated with the study of process. For example, the liver consists of liver cells that are arranged around ducts for transporting bile salts, amongst other products, to the intestine. This refers to structure. Some of the products of digestion are circulated through the liver and transformed by the liver cells into new chemical products important for metabolic processes. This refers to process. Liver cells consist of organelles, that are constructed out of complex proteins, made up in turn of simple molecules, that consists of atomic particles, and so on. This refers to hierarchy. It is the relationship between these components that make the functioning of the liver possible, since function only has relevance in terms of the body as a whole. This means that the liver may be observed as a detoxifying organ, a glucose producing and storing organ, and so forth. These are emergent properties, and the property selected for observation is a design choice.

In short, to gain understanding of the function of a system requires an understanding of the whole of which the system is part, in other words, requires synthetic thinking.

Stability

Geoffrey Vickers (1984) defined a system as a *regulated* set of *relationships*, and the key to its understanding it is the way in which it is regulated. This definition subtly changes the emphasis of understanding to the *relationships* between the components of systems and the *stability* that they show over time.

Regulation (control) therefore, refers to those processes that keep the relationships in the system standing together (stable) over time (Strümpfer, 1992). Contrary to what we believe, it is not *change* that has to be explained in uncertain environments, but *stability*. In other words those factors that keep a system stable (resist entropy) in the face of constant pressure towards disorder. The regulation of relationships in human activity systems was of particular interest to Vickers and will be discussed more fully in a later chapter.

We are usually unaware of the relationships that regulate or keep a system stable, unless the system malfunctions, usually indicating a breakdown in regulation (equilibration is no longer possible). For example, when someone presents with an infection, the fundamental defect is a breakdown of the immune system. Physicians are traditionally taught to attack such a problem by analysis and linear cause and effect. Science and technology enables them to get away with such a simplistic intervention in most cases, but often, that is not enough. Understanding of physiological and patophysiological processes and function is then not sufficient to solve the dilemma, it requires an understanding of what kept the system stable in the first place. To reiterate what Vickers said, it is not disorder that needs explanation, but stability, a position that is more pertinently expressed in the approach in psychology called *salutogenesis* (Manganyi et al, 1993). This approach is not concerned with why people become ill, but instead, why they manage to stay well in a hostile environment.

It is sometimes useful to treat the regulator as a system on its own in order to simplify the problem for the inquirer, but caution is in order since the idea of a regulator separate from the system it regulates is like considering a body without a brain, they inextricably intertwined and cannot be separated in reality. The purpose of this manoeuvre is to apply analysis, modeling, and synthesis, in turn, to the regulatory component of the system inquired into. Furthermore, it is important when doing so to understand that regulatory systems depend on information, and therefore signals, as a necessary requirement for a response. Expansionistic thinking implies an ability to stand back and look at the whole, but more importantly, at the dynamic nature, or ongoing processes of the whole. Hence, it is form of synthetic thinking on a mega-level.

But, we are still left with the question; what are we looking for? We already know that a system consists of structure, process and functional relationships, of which structure by definition does not change over time (is static). Hence, what is of interest here then are (the dynamic) process-function relationships that describe some aspect of the behavior of the system. For example, temperature and blood pressure would be two such descriptors in a living body system, and employee morale and unit production examples of descriptors for a factory as an organizational system. We know that body temperature alters from moment to moment in response to the influence of other components of the body system (rate of metabolism, physical activity, and so on), as well as the body's environment (air temperature, air movement, location, and so on). An understanding of the active relationships between these factors may manifest itself in an understanding of the regulation of body temperature. The aspect of behavior (descriptor) selected for further inquiry is a design choice of the planner and therefore needs careful consideration.

An understanding of system stability may result in "wisdom" about the system, using the following method:

i. Define descriptor variables that are relevant to the phenomenon the planner is trying to explain.
ii. Plot variables over time to find patterns in behavior. For those descriptor variables showing relatively stable relationships, determine necessary co-producers.
iii. Develop a SD model using the co-producers to explain the observed stability.

Summary

Diagram 4: Systems Perspectives

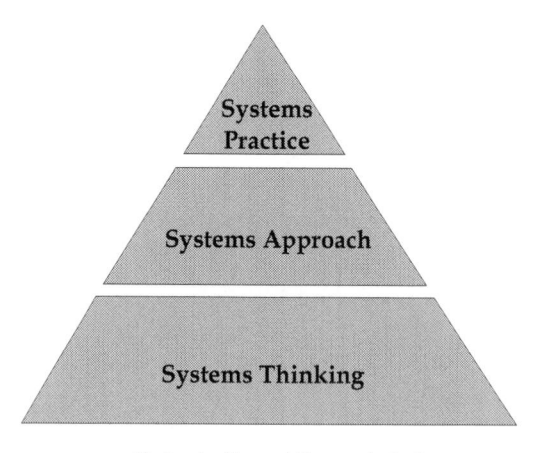

(Strümpfer, Personal Communication)

To summarize then, decision-making in complex unstructured environments may be approached by integrating the three components of the systems idea (see **diagram 4**)[8]. Systems thinking (general systems theory) is a way of thinking about problems in terms of wholes (Checkland, 1991). A *systems approach* (Checkland, 1991) is a methodology that:

---

[8]JP Strümpfer, personal communication.

- Takes a broad view.
- Tries to take all aspects (and viewpoints) into account; and
- Concentrates on the interactions between the different components of the problem.

Systems practice is the application of systems thinking and a systems approach to actively resolve complex poorly structured problem situations.

Table 1: Modes of inquiry

Categories of Knowledge	System Relationships	Systems Practice
Information	Structure	Analysis
Insight	Process	SD modeling
Understanding	Function	Synthesis
"Wisdom"	Regulation	Expansionistic thinking

To gain useful knowledge for decision-making by thinking systemically about complex problems, the following steps are required (compare with **table 1**):

i. Identify the entity under observation as the product of a system, or as part of a larger containing whole.
ii. Use analytical thinking to determine the structure (parts) of the entity or system, in other words, to gain information.
iii. Use synthetic thinking to form an understanding of the external relations (the whole) that the entity is part of and to determine its function in terms of the whole.
iv. Use expansionistic thinking to acquire "wisdom" at a meta-level.

Of all systems, living (biological) systems are the most complex. Living systems in general and human activity systems in particular will be the topic of discussion of the rest of this chapter.

Living Systems

Traditionally, living systems are conceived as machines. This is a legacy of the Cartesian tradition and has had an important influence on approaches to studies in psychiatry and sociology. The belief that human systems are nothing but complex machines is fundamental to the thinking and approach to illness and planning in modern medicine. Mechanical systems are considered to be closed to the environment, and hence, there can be little active exchange of information between the system and its environment. We know today that the belief in the mechanical metaphor is misguided and that living systems are always open systems (Bowler, 1981; Von Bertalanffy, 1968) that depend on interaction with the environment to survive[9]. In other words, they require information about the environment to enable them to act in those ways that may ensure successful adaptation (Buckley, 1967) and survival. Furthermore, an important feature of living systems is that they react *purposefully* to information. Entropy is resisted, and order is maintained in human systems by the active input of *information*.

To maintain the organization (structure) of, and to control living systems, requires the co-operation of subsystems at all levels (Bowler, 1981). Co-operation in turn, depends on input of information about the environment, and more importantly, about other subsystems, in order for the system to adjust. Hence, regulation depends on both the controller (system as a whole) and its components. This has important implications for the way that we conceive human activity systems, as will be shown later.

Information about adjustments made by components is returned to other components of the system. In other words, feedback loops upon which the integrity of the system depends are created. The study of the transfer of information in complex systems and feedback is the interest of the field of cybernetics.

Living systems are constantly exposed to new information that may require a response. A final adjustment (equilibrium) cannot be achieved, and the process of adaptation therefore has no final end point (Bowler, 1981). The result inevitably is an approximation that will have to be adjusted and again and again in time. Systems able to acquire new information about the environment are able to learn, and therefore to adapt more efficiently.

For complex systems to remain viable, some subsystems are needed to perform special (specialized) functions (Bowler, 1981). The more specialized a subsystem becomes, the more dependant it becomes on the system, and in fact, may not be able to survive separately of the system at all. Specialization of subsystems is a response to a need of the system as a whole for specialized components. The more complex a system becomes, the more important the functions vital to survival become, and the less the system can tolerate deviation by subsystems.

---

[9]Humans need external stimuli in order to stay mentally healthy. In fact, sensory deprivation may lead to degeneration of nerve cells in the brain (Berne, 1964). Equilibrium therefore may lead to entropy and may physiologically be an undesirable state for human systems to attain (Von Bertalanffy, 1968).

The next chapter is about human activity systems as the most complex of living systems and most frequently the focus of interest of the systems idea.

Chapter 3: Human Activity Systems

Human activity systems[1], are sets of human activities ordered into wholes, because of some underlying purpose of the participants (Checkland, 1991), and are the products of a man-created universe. Living systems in general are surrounded by, and largely have to deal with a physical universe, but humans, in addition, have to deal with a universe of *symbols* that are created internally by the mind (Von Bertalanffy, 1968)[2].

The ability to intervene in social systems depends critically on the assumptions we make about society. It is fairly generally agreed that most traditional models of society are flawed and very few are of particular practical value. Towards the latter part of his life, Geoffrey Vickers (1894 - 1982)[3] gained respect as a systems and social thinker. He suggested a social theory, based upon systems thinking, that, although not widely known and used, may have the most practical utility of currently available models. His model of appreciation will be used as the fundamental point of departure for thinking about social problems in this text.

Appreciation, according to Vickers, consists of three components (Adams, Catron and Cook in Vickers (1995)).

 i. *Reality judgments*, about what is and is not the case.
 ii. *Value judgments*, about what ought or ought not to be the case; and
 iii. *Instrumental judgments*, about the available means to reduce the mismatch between is and ought.

Vickers (1968) suggests that based upon cybernetic principles there is an ongoing process during which information about both system and environment is compared with internally generated standards, or norms. Any disparity between signal and norm may serve as a trigger for an appropriate response. Appreciation is the process of comparison between the state of the system and the norm.

---

[1]The term human activity system is preferred in this text. The terms sociocultural systems (Buckley, 1967), or social systems (Bowler, 1981), are used by other authors and when used imply the same concept.
[2]The natural sciences study the physical, whereas social science deals with the symbolic part of the human universe (Vickers, 1968; Von Bertalanffy, 196).
[3]Vickers studied classical languages and civilisation at Oxford, and later was influenced by the works of Von Bertalanffy, Wiener, and Ross Ashby. After his retirement in 1955, he devoted all his time to developing and spreading the systems idea. He won the Victoria Cross for bravery on his 21st birthday.

Reality judgments may be influenced by events in the environment, the beliefs of other individuals, and the internal requirements of the individual itself. Individual beliefs are incomplete and inconsistencies are therefore continuously challenged by the environment and other individuals.

Appreciative behavior produces the relations that humans, organizations, or societies attempt to preserve (norms). In open systems, appreciative behavior can never be static, relations are ongoing and norms require adjustment all the time.

Without communication, appreciation cannot take place (because there is no exchange of signals) and norms cannot be adjusted to reflect the reality of a changing environment. Appreciative systems that cannot adapt to a changing world must eventually break down. In Part II, the inability of the health care system to alter its worldview will be shown to be an important contributor to the breakdown of the system. An important reason for this is the inability of those who participate in the system, patients, physicians, health care workers, government and business, to communicate constructively with each other.

Stability

Vickers had a special interest in those factors within human activity systems that ensure stability, which he defined as the continuity of a relation, or set of relations, that are important to us in time (Vickers, 1980). This definition has three implications:

i. That the relationship is continuous (although it does not mean that the system has to last forever)
ii. That the particular relations that are of interest to us is a design choice; and
iii. That the relations are not stable, and hence the product of equilibration at work.

Social systems in the end are constructed out of a web of cultural relationships from which we cannot be separated, and consist of relationships that, because human activity systems are open systems, are changing all the time as a result of the interaction of the participants of the system.

Biological order is innate to our species and change at a rate determined by evolutionary adaptation. *Social* order on the other hand, is a product of culture and therefore our symbolic world varies widely between different cultures and change at a rate dependent on the stability of the social system that it regulates. Order depends on the behavior of the individual members as prescribed by social expectations. Hence, in the end, stability in human activity systems depend on the standards and norms of the system and *trust* that members will behave according to these norms. It is easier to break the trust and discard the norms of a system than to reinstate them and therefore, the protection of trust and norms is important. In addition, their preservation in terms of order requires effort (Second law of thermodynamics), but at the same time order entails the acceptance of constraints and the limits to choice that it induces. Hence, the concept of social stability is inimicable to the notion of individual freedom without constraints.

Diagram 5: Growth and Constraint

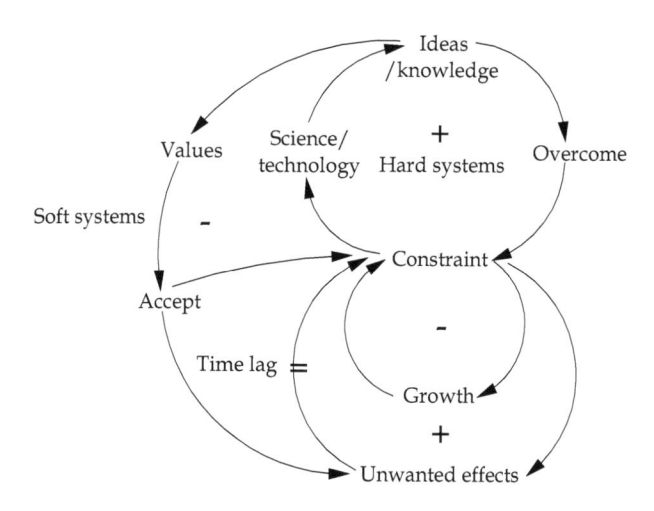

The *regulation* of human activity systems depends on communication and shared systems of interpretation to give it meaning. Social and personal regulation has to do with the setting of standards and norms that are sufficiently consistent, attainable, valid and acceptable to preserve the coherence and stability of societies. Norms and value systems are therefore an integral part of the interpretative systems upon which the stability of communities depends.

All open systems will eventually reach constraints that limit further growth and that act as a restraint on the system (**diagram 5**). Order depends on such processes of *self-regulation*. The system sends out signals and in return receives inputs from the environment that indicates that no further growth or development of the system in that direction is possible. Growth and constraint is balanced by a negative (balancing) feedback loop, in other words, growth takes place until it is restrained, which retards further growth and consequently loosens constraints.

With the advent of Western science and technology (hard systems), it became possible to remove, alter or postpone constraints to growth. Hence we became able to *change* our environment when we received signals indicating constraints. Man was no longer constrained by the laws of nature. However, because of the complexity of natural processes, interference often causes unwanted or unintended side effects such as pollution, over-population, holes in the ozone layer, and so on. These unwanted effects often cause new constraints, not infrequently separated from them in time, hence, they only become noticeable later. In other words, whereas we gained the ability to change and sometimes harness the forces of nature, we lost the ability to control the effects of such changes.[4] This is because we do not understand the necessity of control systems to regulate change. New constraints limit further growth and thus require new solutions to overcome them, in other words, a positive feedback loop is created. This vicious cycle is the result of the myopic worldview of traditional analytic thinking. With synthetic thinking, values and choice are included in decision-making, in other words we may choose to accept the unwanted effects and eventual constraints of machine thinking, or, we may accept the original constraint. More importantly, it is a way of seeking solutions that overcome constraints without creating unwanted effects.

In the archetypal social interaction, human activity was focused on the commune, and was limited either by natural (lack of water, food, and living space), or symbolic constraints (communal norms or values). By contrast, an important result of the new man-made environment is the change from the commune to the organization as the most important area of human social interaction. Hence, the focus shifted from the need to participate toward communal needs for survival, to the wants of the individual (economic man). The resulting rise in the importance of markets as an expression of wants created the belief that the market economy, be it goods, services, or employment, will be self-regulated by the collective values of the *individuals* partaking in it. The belief is that those with access to the market, will create forces of control or regulation, and hence, a belief that whatever the client wants is right as the measure of performance in economical matters. In this way, individuals are supposed to be freed from all constraints so that they may make decisions in whatever way they seem fit, irrespective of the effect it may have on others. This model of free man is fundamental to all

---

[4]Vickers classifies the outcomes of systems intervention as: a) unsuccessful, where the goals of planning was not achieved, b) successful, where the goals were achieved and we are better off, and c) where goals were achieved successfully, but we wish that they had not been. In other words, we are worse off as a result of our success.

emancipatory[5] approaches to the social sciences and depends on the assumption of a high consensus on values, something that does not exist in reality.

Garrett Hardin published a paper in Science in 1968 titled "The tragedy of the commons" (Kauffman, 1980). The problem is illustrated by the free use of grazing on the medieval commons, or village pasture. Individual livestock owners get better off as their herds increase, therefore, since grazing is free, herds are increased as fast as possible. Since all livestock owners argue in the same way, the situation is soon reached where the common resource, grazing, is over used, as a result of which the cattle die and the whole village is worse off. The problem is not helped if individuals elect to reduce their herds, they are individually worse off and furthermore neighbors have an incentive to fill the vacant space. The problem can only be overcome by inviting science or technology to discover a new formula (which will inevitably have new unwanted effects), or by adjusting communal norms or values so that voluntary individual self-alignment of all participants takes place. By accepting the constraints of the system as a whole, the system and all its parts are better off. It is this, the freedom of individuals to choose voluntary self-control to regulate their system of relationships that was of central interest to Vickers.

By considering the whole and the effect of decisions on the whole, we may be able to balance demands to circumvent constraints. Furthermore, decisions about the whole has to include values and hence choice about whether we are prepared to live with current constraints to growth, or with the unwanted effects of measures that will remove them. Soft systems thinking therefore has the capacity to act as a balancing loop to decision-making in a complex environment.

Vickers' Model Of Social Interaction

Humans are communal beings. As a general principle, in human societies there are always more mouths to feed than hands to get and prepare food. The activity of food production and distribution therefore requires a *collective* effort amongst members of a community, as well as some convention to determine the tasks and shares that will be allocated to each participant (Vickers, 1980). The reward for co-operation is the basic individual need satisfaction for food, shelter, protection, and so on that would otherwise be difficult if not impossible.

Different individuals are allocated different tasks to facilitate the efficient achievement of communal goals. These social roles are specialized functions

---

[5]*Emancipate*: to free from restraint, especially legal, social or political (Allen, 1990).

that develop in response to the requirements of communities. The more specialized the role, the more the community (or system) depends on the specialist individual. It is expected of individuals to act out their roles in accordance with communal expectations and their actions are evaluated and interpreted according to the mind map that the commune has of the role. In other words, the community trusts individuals to act out their roles in the fashion determined by communal standards, or *norms*. Without *trust* based upon the belief that individual members of society will act responsibly, the system becomes unstable.

We learn roles and acquire shared norms by observing and following the example of the elders in society. It can be said that we are born into the norms of a culture as a historical product at a particular point in time, since the norms are passed on from generation to generation. We also learn to modify our interpretation of norms in response to pressure from first our elders and later our peers by a process of feedback and adjustment, in other words by *appreciation*.

The individual member, then, by accepting a communal role, benefits from communal efforts but in return has to accept the constraints imposed by communal norms. Hence, participation imposes limitations upon the potential choices that would otherwise be available to the individual member of society. In a well functioning society, constraints are sufficiently flexible to allow individuals to act out their differences without destroying order. Restrictive societies, by disallowing variety, must eventually stagnate as a result of a poverty of ideas. On the other hand, disordered societies in which individuals are allowed a free rein in their choices and actions will inevitable lead to anarchy (entropy). In the end, it is the interaction between individuals and society that ensures social stability.

Responsibility And Norms

The traditional definition of *responsibility*[6] is often understood to mean being answerable to someone else (in the Judeo-Christian ethos often God, the church, or a paternal figure representing authority), and *autonomy*, being answerable to oneself only. Answerability on the whole implies a personal commitment and constraint, just as the concept of responsibility suggests commitment and constraint in a social sense. Commitment and constraint in turn are regulated by internal personal standards (norms) that are used to determine what a person ought to do in a particular circumstance.

---

[6]All quotes in this section, directly or indirectly, are from G. Vickers (1980): Responsibility - Its Sources and Limits, Intersystems Publications.

A more desirable definition of responsibility, for Vickers, would be a state of having accepted a commitment, and of autonomy the right to *select* commitments, the ability to *live* by them, and acceptance of the *constraints* imposed by the commitment. The trouble with modern man is the elevation of individualism at the expense of the community. This is also the dilemma of emancipation, a belief that seeks to *remove* the constraints to individual goal satisfaction (Flood and Jackson, 1991). Both economic and emancipated man therefore has an entropic effect on social stability.

It is a tacit assumption that people will act toward us in a responsible way. At the same time, our own norms are made explicit to others by the way we act, or conduct ourselves. It is shared norms that enable social structures to hang together, hence the importance that we shall be able to *trust* others to act in a responsible way. Shared standards and norms are often codified by society in laws and regulations, to enforce responsible behavior and stability.

Human societies are constantly in evolving and may therefore be classified as open systems. Hence, the norms that regulate communal life are constantly challenged to change in response to new signals from the environment. The standards (or mental ideas) tend to resist change in an effort to seek order and stability, but a measure of disorder is desirable to ensure viability in the face of a constantly changing environment. It is possible to conceive of this tension between stability and the necessity for change as the polar opposites in a process of equilibration.

Modern Man

According to Vickers, the ascent of modern man may be traced to around 1776 based upon Adam Smith's (1723 - 1790) concept of free markets, Jeremy Bentham's (1748 - 1832) philosophy of utilitarianism, and the American Declaration of Independence (1776).[7]

The ideal of utilitarianism is based upon a belief in the greatest happiness for the greatest number. Logically, this found expression in the socialist (and Marxist) faith in the power of legislation to recreate and regulate human social order.

The introduction of Smith's idea of the market economy redefined the criteria for the creation of national wealth as:

- A co-operative enterprise.
- Infinitely expandable; and

---

[7] The 18th Century is also identified as the start of the age of "enlightenment", from which we are gradually emerging (Anderson, 1996).

- The freedom of the individual to exchange labor, goods, services, and so on.

Such a structure can only survive given highly specific socio-political preconditions, namely:

- The sanctity of *contract*, culturally and legally.
- The abolition of all constraints, except those imposed by the market.
- The acceptance of market constraints; and
- A belief that the market will be self-regulating.

Table 2: Social Control

System	Controlled by	Method of Control	Unexpected Outcome
Entrepreneurial	Consumer	Market	Unchecked growth
Political	Voter	Ballot	Power of minorities
Scientific	Peers	Positions, facilities	Decreased predictability
Technological	Markets	Skills, products	Decreased manageability

The market economy expresses itself through science and technology. The original understanding of science had been that of an activity, or skill, comprising both a process and a product. Unfortunately, the modern version impoverished itself by its focus on analysis to the exclusion of cultural context and values. Equally, throughout the ages technology progressed with *"an uncanny ignorance of the scientific principles guiding it"* (Vickers, 1980), in this way doing exactly the same thing, resulting in a false belief in its own power. The scientific-technological environment described here requires a belief in systems controlling themselves in the ways presented in **Table 2**:

The problem with all of the above mentioned systems, are that instead of being self regulating, as was expected, they have been self-exciting in a linear fashion. The unrestrained demand of economic man must inevitably reach some limit to growth, unless it is supported by unlimited resources, something that is impossible in the natural systems upon which science and technology depends. We are now entering an era where many natural systems are probing the limits of the resources on which we depend. The trouble is that the outcome of extravagant demand is in conflict with our ability to satisfy these demands. On the one hand, economic man is the ultimate individualist, and on the other, its self-created world spawned an environment where interdependence is required more than ever before in order to survive.

Vickers (1980) quotes Lynton Caldwell to illustrate the conditions Western society will require to survive the changes affected in the previous century, and I would like to repeat the quote verbatim.

"The emphasis on popular rights needs to shift towards social responsibilities by which alone such rights can be created and maintained. Autonomous egoism should give place to a sense of organic interdependence. Progressive expansion should make way for an ideal of self-sustaining growth. Economic imperatives should give way to ecological imperatives. Technological imperatives should be subordinated to judgments of political need. External constraints which invite efforts to overcome them should give way to self-imposed restraints, supported by a sense of personal commitment to accept them."

The major obstacles to the acceptance of these principles are self-erected cultural barriers.

The difficulty in controlling human affairs is in selecting constraints and then generating sufficient agreement to ensure that they are accepted as regulators for the required action.

Models Of Organization

A feature of human systems is that individuals may participate in a number of systems at the same time. Some may be organized vertically as part of a hierarchy, and others horizontally. For example, a school may be conceived as a physical system (organization), that is part of a number of other physical systems, such as water systems, sewerage systems, electrical power systems, and so on. At the same time it is also a social system that partakes in other human activities, such as education, finance, administration, and so forth, that each may be conceptualized as separate systems. Hence, in a school as a system and organization (much the same as in other human activity systems), demands may be made on both pupils and teachers by a number of intimately related systems at the same time. The implication is that the boundary of an inquiry into any of these systems is an arbitrary one for the purpose of the inquiry and does not reflect realistically the interconnectedness that cannot be separated.

Table 3: Purposeful behavior in organizations.

Type of organization	Components	System	Containing System
Mechanismic	None	None	Purposeful
Organismic	None	Purposeful	Purposeful
Social system	Purposeful	Purposeful	Purposeful

Russell Ackoff (1981) developed a model that is useful for interpreting the way that human activity systems are organized. This model consists of the following (**table 3**):

- *Mechanismically* conceived organizations.
- *Organismically* conceived organizations.
- The organization conceived as a *social system*.

The Cartesian worldview was referred to earlier. This view led to a concept of the universe as a clock or machine that consists of parts and interactions that can be analyzed by reduction. This is the mechanistic view[8]. In mechanismic systems, both components and systems as a whole are considered not to have purposes of their own. The purpose of organizations as machines is to provide their creators with an adequate return on their investments, in other words, to produce a profit. Hence, the purpose of such systems is determined by the containing systems of which they are part. Furthermore, workers are considered to be components of the machine (the organization) and their personal objectives are consequently irrelevant. In this model there is an emphasis on the efficiency of the parts and on external control (Flood and Jackson, 1991).

The introduction of the concept of cybernetics led to a view of the organization as an organism[9]. In this metaphor, the purpose of the organization is survival and growth and profits are a necessity for survival. Management is the brain of the organism and as such has to accept full responsibility for the organization. The well being of the workers now becomes the concern of the organization, but this does not include an interest in their personal needs. The organization receives inputs from its environment and dispenses outputs back into it. Similarly, management receives information from the different sections in the organization and sends back outputs as instructions. There is therefore an emphasis on the flow of information. In organismic systems, the system as a whole has a purpose, as does the larger systems within which it is contained, but the components are conceived to be without purposes of their own, and hence the need for their control by management.

These metaphors are now being replaced by the concept of the organization as a social system (Von Bertalanffy, 1968). This implies an organization that:

- Is a purposeful system in its own right
- Is itself part of one or more other purposeful systems; and
- Consist of parts (people) that have purposes of their own.

---

[8]The mechanismic metaphor is inherent to all hard systems.
[9]This is the operative metaphor of living systems theory and other cybernetic approaches.

The functioning of such an organization depends upon the interaction between itself and the people it consists of, as well as between itself and the other systems of which it is a part. In such a model, the actions of the organization have effects at many different levels, since it is part of a complex social system. The problem of management now becomes one of integrating the purposes of the organization with that of its employees, and also with the systems that it is part of, to ensure optimal function. These purposes are often at odds with each other and the key to stability is successful co-operation. The social organization is the metaphor most consistent with a systems approach.

Another useful metaphor is the *political metaphor* described by Flood and Jackson (1991). Here the emphasis is on competition and the pursuit of power between groups (and individuals). The character of such organizations may be unitary (common objectives between members), pluralist (diverging group interests), or coercive (oppositional and contradictory interests). This metaphor is common in political systems.

Control[10]

Inherent to all metaphors of organization is the problem of *control*[11]. The underlying assumption in mechanismic organizations is that control is at the level of environmental inputs. Once the input enters the system, the flow can be controlled in a predetermined manner. In other words, it is possible to guide the inputs in the system by a set of specifications. Control is therefore external to the system and static.

In the organismic metaphor, the locus of control is the flow of information. The brain, or management, receives an input of information in response to which it sends out information about the objectives that it had decided upon. Consequently, there is an emphasis on the measurement of performance and the co-ordination of actions. Control is internal to the system.

In the organization as a social system *aligned self-control* replaces control. The emphasis is on a shared understanding by all the participants of the purpose of the system, and the context within which it operates. An understanding of the *vision*[12] of an organization ensures participation and enables the participants to act in a coordinated way by self-control. The emphasis is on

---

[10]Strümpfer (1994a)
[11]*Control*: the power to direct, or command; a means of restraint. *Command*: to have authority or control over (Allen, 1992).
[12]*Vision*: a statement of where we want to go and what we will be like when we get there. In other words, it is a picture of the future you seek to create for yourself (Senge, 1994). This is very similar to an ideal as an objective.

vision, alignment,[13] and empowerment, and the processes necessary to achieve it. In principle, there is very little difference between aligned self-control and Vickers' concept of responsibility. Both entail a personal commitment to contribute towards fulfilling the purpose of the system for the common good and co-operation.

Both the mechanismic and organismic models assume a linear model of causality, which imply that it is possible for a person or persons to control resources and variables in order to produce a particular output. The organization as social system is designed on the basis of a multiple causality model, within which it is impossible to be in complete control. The concept of individual responsibility within such a system has no meaning.

Causality In Complex Systems

According to the popular image of science, everything is in principle predictable and controllable (Bateson, 1979). If this is not the case, it will become possible when we acquire more knowledge. This perception is based upon the Cartesian system, which has three rules:

i. Never accept anything as true that cannot clearly be shown to be true.
ii. Divide every problem into as many parts as necessary to adequately explain it.
iii. To reason logically, start with the simplest known facts and assemble them into more complex entities (fact nets).

This (reductionist) approach is the cause of two assumptions upon which the image of science is based, namely:

i. Knowledge is finite and if we can identify the simplest truths, it is conceptually possible to collect all possible knowledge in the universe and in time to construct it into an interconnected whole.
ii. The collection of knowledge is a sequential linear process (Bateson, 1979).

These assumptions are basic to the linear cause and effect model that has been used very successfully in modern science. This, the deterministic system, is the dominant view of causality in Western science and technology (Feinstein, 1988).

---

[13]*Alignment*: when a group of people function together as a whole (Senge, 1990). Unaligned groups may work very hard, but their efforts are at cross-purpose, and therefore inefficient.

The modern concept of causation begins with David Hume. According to him, when two objects are constantly observed to occur together, one can be inferred to be the cause of the other (Russell, 1993). The problem is that no matter how many times such a connection is observed, it is still impossible to be absolutely certain that the association will be observed the next time it occurs. Hence, in the end, causality is based upon a *belief* that the occurrence will take place, but this belief cannot be proven beyond doubt. In other words, we experience sensations that are then ordered by the mind, hence, causality is the product of an association of ideas (Tamas, 1991). On the basis of this argument, Russell concludes that causal laws in the physical sciences are merely inferences about the observed course of nature.

Immanuel Kant reasoned that causality is an apriori assumption, together with mathematics, and the concepts of space and time, the latter being a necessary condition for any meaningful human observation to take place. According to Kant, the outer world causes that which can be observed empirically and we then mentally order these observations in time and space (Russell, 1993; Tamas, 1991). This approach to causality implies the use of a system of induction.

J.S. Mill framed four canons of inductive method, which can be usefully employed by assuming the laws of causality based upon Hume and Kant's reasoning (Russell, 1993). The canons have been the basis for the scientific method used in researching medical problems in particular. Of particular importance is the Fifth canon, which assumes a causal connection if an associated *variation* can be shown between two events (Churchman and Ackoff, 1950). This method is widely used in medical research, but neither a necessary nor sufficient condition needs to be established between the two events.

The basis of linear causality is "if...then" logic. For causality to exist, the cause has to be both necessary and sufficient for the effect to take place (Ackoff, 1981). One object under investigation is the cause of another object under investigation (its effect), if both objects belong to the same natural mechanical system, and the first object precedes the second in time (Ackoff and Emery, 1972).

At the end of World War II, the notion developed that causality in complex systems may be circular rather than linear (Bateson, 1979). The concept of circular causality underwent further development in the field of cybernetics, and as system dynamics in the systems community (Flood and Jackson, 1991). It means that a producer produces a product that will be the producer of another product and so on, in a recursive manner[14]. Circular causality, or feedback loops, implies that every element is both cause and effect at the same time. Two kinds of causal loops can be identified (Senge et al., 1994; Senge, 1990):

Diagram 6: Feedback

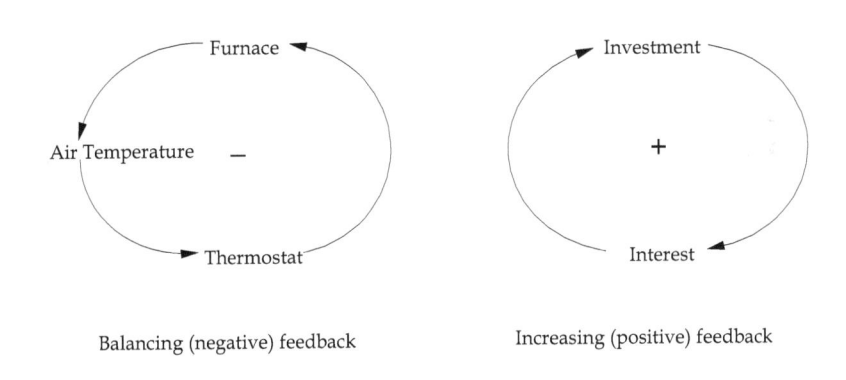

```
         Furnace                          Investment
   Air Temperature    −                        +
         Thermostat                       Interest

   Balancing (negative) feedback   Increasing (positive) feedback
```

i. *Reinforcing* (positive feedback) loops that lead to amplified growth or decline.
ii. *Balancing* (negative feedback) loops that limit growth.

The simplest example of a balancing loop is that of a heating system (see **diagram 6**). A room is heated by a furnace, which elevates air temperature that is detected by a thermostat, which shuts off the furnace when it gets too hot. This causes a drop in air temperature, the thermostat turns the furnace on again, and so on.

Examples of reinforcing feedback loops are compound interest and the growth of cancerous cells. Two or more loops may interact and balance each other. The control of animal populations is an example of two feedback loops balancing each other (**diagram 7**).

If there is a large number of prey, there is more food for predators, which increase in number, causing a reduction in numbers of prey, less food and therefore fewer predators. As the predators increase in number, there is less

---

[14]Bateson (1979) credits Rosenblueth, Wiener, and Bigelow for proposing the self-correcting circuit and its variants.

prey, more food and when the number of predators decline, the number of prey increases.

Diagram 7: Animal Populations

(Adapted with permission from the author from:
DL Kauffman (1980) *Systems I. An Introduction to Systems Thinking*)

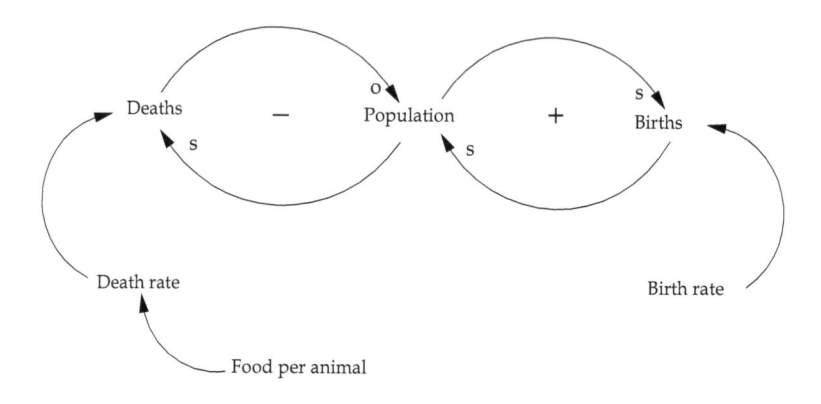

```
         o                        s
Deaths  ─  Population    +     Births
   s              s
Death rate                  Birth rate
        Food per animal
```

When applied to complex systems with many interactions, models with multiple causal loops (a system dynamics model) can be developed (see for example **diagram 8**). This creates a powerful method for perceiving:

- *Interrelationships*; and
- Processes of *change* in complex systems.

The advantage of such an approach is that hidden causes of problem situations are exposed and that an idea may be formed of the possible effects of any intended changes to the system.

A system dynamics model is the only reasonable model available at present for understanding the causal interactions of complex systems. Furthermore, the model is of particular relevance to the understanding of the way that human interactions are structured, which in turn is fundamental to their regulation. It is important to understand that this model does not exclude linear models of causality.

These linear and circular concepts of causality were challenged by Edgar Singer, who proposed a producer-product model of causality instead. According to his model, no individual producer is ever sufficient to produce a product, hence every product has at least one co-producer. In other words, the producer is necessary for the product but not sufficient. The emphasis is on the *relationships* between the parts of the object under investigation, rather than the object individually. To identify all co-producers, the possible contribution of all aspects in the environment of the problem has to be considered when an attempt is made to determine causality (Ackoff, 1981), hence a broad view has to be taken. Furthermore, a single producer may have a number of different products and different products may have the same producers. This model has particular relevance for the study of complex systems.

Diagram 8: Complex Causal Systems

(Adapted with permission from the author from:
DL Kauffman (1980) *Systems I. An Introduction to Systems Thinking*)

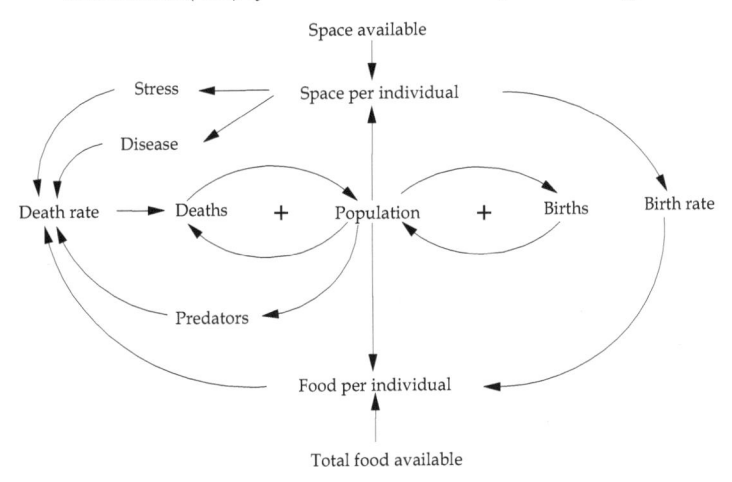

Power Interactions

In a significant number of human interactions, power relationships are at work (Checkland, 1991; Checkland and Scholes, 1991; Vickers, 1972). Power is most often defined as the ability to unilaterally and unidirectionally cause the outcomes one wishes (Simon in Torbert (1991)). In a social sense, this means that the emotions or behavior of other people will be affected (Boulding, 1987; Winter, 1973). Power interactions may take place on an individual or a group level. In the latter instance, people tend to gather around communal issues[15] (form *polis*[16]), which may lead to competition and often to the pursuit of power (Ackoff, 1981; Boulding, 1987; Checkland and

---

[15]This is Churchman's (1979) definition of politics.
[16]An essential part of *polis* is the creation of shared images (Churchman, 1979).

Scholes, 1991; Vickers, 1972). This of course is what is meant by Flood and Jackson's (1991) political metaphor referred to earlier. Politics is the source of conflict in organizations and frustration to planners.

Types of power

Those that hold power control, or attempt to control, the means that others need to satisfy the ends they desire. The concept of power therefore assumes some form of control. Control here is conceived as giving direction to, or governing (Strümpfer, 1994a). According to Toffler (1990), control over the sources of coercion (by the threat of violence), money, and knowledge, confers power. This is a restricted view of power via the control of resources. Torbert (1991) takes a broader view, similar to the power relationships described by Flood and Jackson (1991). Torbert classifies power relationships into:

- *Unilateral* power, where the individual *yields* power to a stronger entity for protection against violence or the threat of violence.
- *Diplomatic* power, where power is generated by the power-yielder (the power of the weak). In this instance, leadership takes place by diplomacy and consensus.
- *Rational* power, where power comes from acting rationally and ethically, rather than being forced from the outside to do so. In other words, acting in ways where we treat others and ourselves as ends, rather than means.
- *Integrating* power, where all the foregoing is integrated into a single entity. This kind of power only has meaning when those in power consciously reflect upon the use of their power. It is this form of power that is of particular interest to systems thinking.

Table 4: A comparison of Torbert's and Flood and Jackson's concepts of power

Torbert	Flood and Jackson
Unilateral power	Coercive power
Diplomatic power	Pluralist power
Rational power	Unilateral
Integrating power	None

Flood and Jackson's coercive power is recognized by rivalry and contradictory interests, pluralist power by diverging group interests that are held together by a loose coalition, and unitary power by common objectives. The amount of conflict in groups decreases on a scale from coercive to unitary power. According to Flood and Jackson's (1991) TSI model, there is no systems methodology currently available to solve the dilemma of coercive power, but Ulrich's critical systems heuristics (CSH) may be useful for dealing with other power relationships. An important aspect of Ulrich's CSH is the dialectic between what is (reality) and what ought to be (ethics and morality) (see also Vickers' appreciation). This is based upon Churchman's design of inquiring systems, which will be discussed later on. In this model, Kant contributes to reason through the dialectic between what is and what ought to be done (Ulrich, 1994b),[17] and Singer the concept of ideals, as shall be seen later.

Diagram 9: Power Interactions

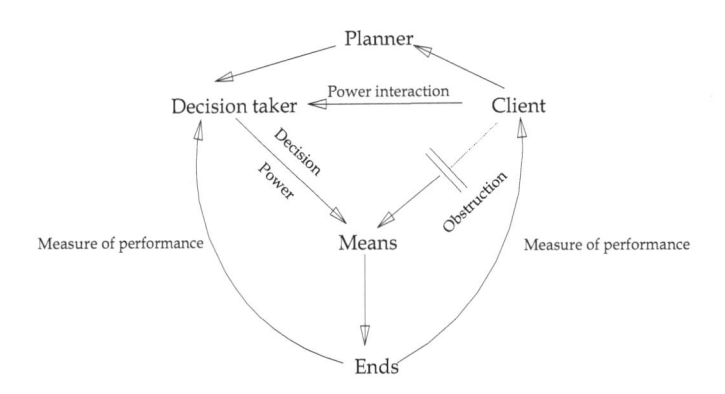

Unilateral or diplomatic power is the most commonly used forms of power. The dialectic opposite would be integrative power, which is an ideal, and a more ethical and just use of power.

The power motive (see diagram 9)

Churchman's (1971) method of planning suggests three roles that will influence planning and the outcomes of planning. They are:

- The *planner*.
- The *client*[18], or entity that benefits from planning.

---

[17] According to Kant, reason is either *theoretical* and produces understanding of what is, or *practical*, which helps to determine what ought to be done (Ulrich, 1994). This is similar to the judgment of fact (reality judgments) and judgment of significance (value judgments) of Vickers' (1984) concept of appreciation.
[18] Strümpfer makes a distinction between the client, the designed beneficiary of planning, and the beneficiary, or someone that benefits from planning but was not expected to do so.

- The *decision maker*[19], who controls the means to implement planning, in other words is a source of power.

The client is someone who acts purposefully, and has a number of possible futures with a preference for some over the others (Churchman, 1971). Churchman follows Singer's concept of purpose, proposing that humans seek goals, as well as the power for attaining them. In terms of this model, power is derived from available means, knowledge of the appropriate means to select, and co-operation with others with similar goals (Churchman, 1979). Purpose can be a goal (short-term objectives), an objective (medium term objectives), or an ideal (which can be approached forever, but never attained).

The decision maker controls the means that will be necessary to achieve the desired ends of the client. Hence, the decision taker has the power to satisfy the client's ends. For clients to satisfy their ends, they have to find not only the means to do so, but also the entity that controls the means. The decision taker is in a position to determine the outcome of the client's objectives and the interaction therefore by definition constitutes a power relationship. On the other hand, the decision taker in turn is constrained by an environment, which limits the use of power.

The implication of this interaction is that one of the planner's roles, which neither Churchman nor Ulrich makes explicit, is to act as facilitator between client and decision taker. Hence, planners attempt to integrate the mind maps of clients and decision takers. This is a core concept of group learning. The difficulty of course is that a single entity may play more than one role in the interaction, or even all three roles at the same time. The source of power and the implications of its use are of critical importance to design, but more importantly, implementation of planning.

The strength of Ulrich's CSH in addressing power relationships is that it makes these relationships explicit through conscious reflection. The problem with coercive power is not in its nature, but in the fact that such structures are often unable or unwilling to reflect on the implications of their position and actions. It is unlikely that any methodology, systems or otherwise, will ever be able to resolve coercive power, other than through the barrel of a gun. However, in the case of unitary or pluralist relationships, the nature of the interaction is such that conscious reflection and therefore intervention becomes possible.

---

[19]Strümpfer distinguishes between the decision taker, the entity that makes the decision, and decision maker, who may help to shape the decision, but does not have decision-making authority.

Who holds power?

The role of the decision taker, and more importantly, the motivation for being in a position of power is a highly complex behavioral issue when individual power is considered. It becomes even more so when the source of power is situated in a group. Winter argues that the power motive[20] of individuals is a disposition to strive for particular goals. Those individuals who strive for power have power as their goal. However, not all individuals have power per se as the ultimate goal. To many, power is necessary for need fulfillment in a broader sense, in other words to achieve a particular purpose.

In groups, such as organizations, power tends to be hierarchical, in other words there usually is a higher authority that is in a position to overturn a decision made at a lower level. This hierarchy is often related to the concepts of responsibility, authority[21] and control, which in turn are closely related to the image of power. If something goes wrong, the question usually is: Who is responsible? According to Senge (1990), a political environment is one in which "who" is more important than "what". Consequently, the best decision is the one that keeps the individual politically powerful (Churchman, 1971).

Organizations tend to be either authoritarian or democratic. In the former, members expect subordination to higher, and authority over lower roles. Decisions are made by higher roles and transmitted down the chain of command. Feedback of information takes place if requested by higher roles (Boulding, 1987). This is in effect what happens in a mechanismically conceived organization (Ackoff, 1981) and the power expressed is of a coercive kind. Democratic organizations also feature higher and lower roles, but authority is supposed to proceed from lower to higher roles. Decisions are made by those in higher roles by discussion and modified by feedback from lower roles (Boulding, 1987). This is the power relationship of an organismically conceived organization (Ackoff, 1981). Democratic organizations with inadequate leadership are unstable. This is usually the result of a difference in goals (norms) as perceived by leadership as opposed to the rest of the organization.

Polis forms around particular issues or goals, and usually dissolves or reform around new issues when the goal is attained. If unsuccessful, they may survive for a very long time or eventually disappear. They usually have no concept of progress, nor do they have a measure of performance

---

[20]Motive in this environment is understood to be the purposeful behaviour of individuals.
[21]According to Winter (1973), the English word power is derived from the Latin root *potere*, which means to be able to. Authority therefore is to be able to act independently (Allen, 1992).

(Churchman, 1971). Organized structures also form images of the roles of those involved with them. Every organization therefore assumes some form of power structure and relationship. These roles tend to influence and in turn are influenced by those who hold them. Hence, power roles as well as power relationships are continuously changing.

The acquisition of power

Winter (1973) describes three dimensions of power.

- The relative inequality of status or strength between two entities. (A is in a position of strength relative to B).
- Legitimacy or moral force. Legitimate or moral power is often referred to as authority or command. This kind of power enables those with lesser strength or status. (The power of the weak).
- The force with which those with more strength and status resist the intentions of those with less strength and status.

The ability to be in a position of power (be a leader) is determined mostly by situational factors. Those that have been identified as significant are:

- Certain positions.
- Socio-economic status.
- Personality characteristics of group members.
- Size and degree of organization of the group.
- The nature of the task.

In general, if a group is allowed to elect a leader, the purpose of and resources available to the group will determine the choice. Those perceived to be in a position to facilitate the achievement of group ends will be elected as leaders and the group will perceive their success in terms of the success with which they are able to achieve these ends. The way the group perceives leaders may change when the goals of the group change. On the other hand, individuals who seek power in order to satisfy their own ends may influence the perceptions and goals of the group. In other words, such individuals will attempt to align collective objectives with individual personal goals.

Kirton (1989) described the effect of preferred creative styles in decision-making. Creative styles may range from innovators, who are high in creativity and prefer to change systems, to adaptors, who prefer implementation and therefore to improve systems. There are early indications that preferred creative style might have an important effect on dominance and therefore leadership style. All social communities have members who tend to be dominant (α-individuals), and who others who are not (ß-individuals). According to Gibb (quoted by Van der Molen (1989)), two opposite forms of dominance exists, namely leadership, where authority is spontaneously accorded by fellow group members, and domination, where authority derives from power apart from the group. It would appear as if creative α-individuals tend to lead autocratically and innovative α-individuals by consensus. Innovative α-individuals who cannot lead tend to integrate poorly into social groups and become outcasts (ω-individuals)[22].

The composition of personnel in organizations tends to change cyclically. A cycle starts when there is a need for innovation to ensure the survival of the organization. During this period innovators are likely to be in the majority. Leadership during this period is more likely to be by a creator and therefore autocratic. However, innovators tend to be poor implementers and the number of the latter must eventually increase in order to achieve desired ends. Leadership then is more likely to become consensual[23]. Eventually, there will be a majority of adaptors, decreased innovation, stagnation, and the cycle repeats. Hence, it would be natural for leadership style and therefore power relationships to change in organizations, depending on the collective needs of the organization at a given point in time.

Ethical power

One can conclude from the discussion so far, that power relationships are highly complex and also constantly evolving (changing). Furthermore, at different times an organization may have different power needs. From the foregoing discussion, an important recurring theme is the concept of control. Hence, underlying assumptions about control influences power, the perception of power, and the use of power.

Most models of control assume the reductionistic linear cause and effect model of Western science. This is typical of authoritarian and democratic power systems. However, complex systems in general and human systems in particular are governed by the laws of non-linear causality, with feedback loops, complex multiple interactions, and time lags. Control and the use of power therefore take place within a complex environment over which less control than naturally assumed exists.

A model of control based upon the latter is that of aligned self-control. This model assumes a shared understanding of the context within which the system operates, and a shared vision of the objectives of the system. The shared understanding and vision enables the parts of the system to interact

---

[22]See for example Wilson (1967) for a discussion of such individuals and their interaction with society.
[23]These two styles of leadership represent Torbert's diplomatic and unilateral metaphors of power.

synergistically. Hence, the behavior of individual parts is under their own control. This has important implications for an ethical concept of power.

Participation is vital for ensuring a collective understanding and vision. Without participation, aligned self-control would not be possible. The process of participation necessarily involves the concepts of group learning, namely the questioning of assumptions upon which decisions are made. In this sense, reflection about power issues is a necessity and may ensure the ethical use of power. The fact is that the use of power cannot take place, unless the wishes and interests of those who will be affected by it are taken into consideration (Vickers, 1972). Any action taken will affect someone other than the decision taker. This is an important collateral of the use of power, since it involves the question of whether the use of power will ensure betterment (guarantee a favorable outcome).

In terms of Kant's dialectical concept of reason and Vickers' model of appreciation referred to before, power relationships on the one hand consists of the reality of what can be observed, and on the other of the (neglected) freedom to use power in a way to improve social systems. The former is the reality of unilateral and democratic power and the latter the attempt to achieve betterment by the use of power as described above.

Because unilateral and diplomatic models of power assume control within a simple causal system, the use of this kind of power often has unforeseen results in increasingly complex social environments. Power of this kind is what Churchman calls the enemy of the systems approach. The fact that they are still the most prevalent forms in use is an indication of the inability of systems planners to influence those in power to reflect upon and use a more ethical approach. Furthermore, the reality is that until personal growth has taken place to modify the behavior of those exercising this kind of power, this kind of power relationship will be part of the environment that the planner cannot alter.

Individuals respond to power interactions by fight, flight, or verbal negotiation (Smith, 1989). The first two are primitive responses and if the latter fails, the response is often passive flight or passive aggression. In this way, coerced individuals find many punitive ways for making the implementation of unpopular decisions impossible. Individual co-operation therefore, in the end, can only be ensured through successful negotiation and therefore participation.

The development of Torbert's integrating power in individuals can only take place by a process of personal understanding and growth. This process is based on the concept of a just society as described by Rawls (Torbert, 1991). The moral use of unilateral power can only take place if; just rules are made, the rules are explained in an understandable way, and the rules apply equally to those who enact them. In a just society, diplomatic power takes place within the context of group goals and norms. The personal experience of the morality of authority and association leads to an association with the principles of justice behind the rules and a rational understanding of the principles of justice[24]. This then is integrated power. This position is similar to Vickers' (1972) concept of democratic consensus.

Democratic consensus has limitations. In a democratic system, those who dissent must agree to implement the decision of the majority, while the latter must tolerate a continuance of debate. Therefore, liberty means to keep man the doer in the service of man the done-by, without frustrating either party in the process. This places an increasing responsibility on both. Beliefs about the nature of the political situation, the goals of political power and the mode of political action are shared by both doers and done-by. These beliefs are created and altered by democratic dialogue and at times require radical questioning and innovation.

Purposeful Behavior

An important feature of human activity systems is the fact that humans act purposefully. Ackoff (1981) understands purpose to mean the ability to select one's own objectives (ends) and the means (actions) for pursuing them. Objectives and means are selected by a process of inquiry that leads to choice. Preferences for particular means and ends, as well as available knowledge, are the parameters used to make informed decisions. Ends that may be pursued are:

- *Goals*: Desirable objectives that may be obtained within a specific time limit.
- *Objectives*: Desirable outcomes that will not be attained within a particular period of time, but may be attained later.
- *Ideals*: Desirable outcomes that can never be attained, but progress can be made indefinitely towards the ideal.

The selection of desirable objectives is a product of our internal symbolic world. The fulfillment of wants may be constrained either by our natural environment, or by the symbolic environment created by others or ourselves. Hard systems methodologies are useful for dealing with the former and soft systems methodologies with the latter.

---

[24]Rawls' concept of justice is based upon a system of basic equal liberty (in the Kantian sense), and an agreement that inequality of position and wealth will only be tolerated as long as it benefits those with less. See also the earlier discussion of Vickers' work.

The selection of ends, in particular, is of importance, since values or ethics ought to be included in the decision-making process. It is in this area that systems thinking has particular merit.

Reason

A fundamental difference between humans and other living organisms is the fact that we are *conscious*[25] of both ourselves as individuals, and of our environment (Checkland, 1991). As a result of this, we have the ability for abstract reasoning, and on the basis of this the freedom to select our own actions (act purposefully). In other words, humans are able to construct possible future events before they happen (plan and make predictions), and on the basis of this to select possible courses of action. Decisions made in response to a changing environment are often made in an *intuitive* way, but because of our awareness[26] we are able to use *reason*[27] to make better decisions. Reason is a powerful tool when it is used for testing the underlying assumptions upon which our decision-making is actually based. We can therefore use reason to inquire into the processes by which we make decisions and through a process of inquiry can learn about the way that we arrive at our decisions. In this way, we can learn to make better decisions.

In order to survive in an uncertain and constantly changing environment, we have to observe events in the environment and save our experiences in memory, in other words, we must be able to *learn*[28]. These experiences are images of life as we have experienced or perceived them. They are useful for avoiding previous mistakes, or re-enacting past successes when situations similar to those experienced in the past are encountered. Our survival (and the survival of complex systems) depends on the ability to use knowledge to adapt and learn. The term survival is used here in the sense of being able to maintain stability in an unstable environment.

Mind maps are constructed when information about the environment is internally transformed into knowledge. Knowledge in turn may be adjusted in response to experience, in which case learning takes place. In addition,

---

[25]Kaplan and Sadock (1991) define *consciousness* as a state of awareness, including both apperception (perception modified by one's own emotions and thoughts) and sensorium (state of functioning of the special senses).
[26]*Awareness* is the process by which information in the brain is made globally available to motor processes such as speech and bodily action (Chalmers, 1995).
[27]*Reasoning* is the ability to connect ideas consciously, coherently, and purposively (Runes, 1963).
[28]*Learning* is the process whereby knowledge is created by the transformation of experience (Kolb, 1984). Or, learning is an increase in the degree of knowledge or understanding over time (Ackoff and Emery, 1972).

knowledge may be used for conscious decision-making by mentally constructing possible outcomes of actions. Such decision-making is useful for purposeful action. Of central concern to any decision-making therefore are the questions, how did we acquire knowledge, and, how do we verify the validity of this knowledge? This will be the focus of discussion of the next chapter.

Chapter 4: Knowledge About Complex Phenomena

The structure of knowledge is represented by the net of facts that society preserves as cultural images of life, often in the written word. This knowledge is constantly challenged and may change during the process of learning. In addition, knowledge acquires function or purpose when it is used for inquiry into the questions about life that humans constantly try to resolve. To understand the regulation of knowledge requires an understanding of the relationship between knowledge and human activity systems.

What Is Knowledge?

Data may be considered as a convenient way to store and transfer bits of information, and when joined together in specific contexts, becomes known as information (Kock, McQueen and Baker, 1996). For example, the letters of the alphabet are bits, which combined in strings become words, in other words information. The meaning of information depends on the context within which collections of data are used. Not only does the way that words are strung together in sentences confer meaning, but also the meaning depends on the context within which they are used. For example, the word "power" has different meanings that are contextually dependant; it may be used to mean the ability to act, authority, physical strength, in physics the rate of energy output, etc.

Knowledge results when the implications of available information are consciously understood. The context of knowledge may be altered by experience and when this happens, learning takes place. Knowledge forms the basis upon which decisions are made about a changing environment.

There was a time when the total body of knowledge known to man was limited enough for one individual to know almost all of it. Consequently, it was possible for early man to retain much of what was known in memory. Later, this knowledge was printed in textbooks, and by studying the texts, a person could know most of what constituted current knowledge at the time. Furthermore, it was possible to keep these texts for reference. Today, the body of knowledge is enormous and a single person cannot hope to know even an infinitesimal amount of available knowledge. To use this knowledge efficiently requires specialization of some kind, but the problem with specialization is tunnel vision, or the worms eye view.

Some systems, such as the health care system, depend on specialized knowledge for their survival. They may acquire more members with special knowledge (specialists) in response to the need for more knowledge in the system. Knowledge workers use their knowledge purposefully to interpret incoming information, and also create knowledge by adjusting existing knowledge through learning. Systems with a large number of knowledge workers may be conceptualized as knowledge systems, most professions being activity systems of this kind. In them, data and information is exchanged between members, instead of goods, or services. The challenge facing such systems is how to make knowledge workers co-operate effectively and efficiently. Inefficient systems have a high degree of entropy and disorder, with members working at cross-purpose to each other. On the other hand, systems in which members co-operate are more ordered and efficient. This, as will be shown later, has specific implications for the health care system, which by definition is a knowledge system.

An implication of the discussion so far, is that knowledge results from the interpretation of information by active personality systems, an interpretation that takes place within the framework of the prior knowledge that is unique to each individual. This may have an important implication for the way we conceptualize learning. Firstly, two or more individuals can never acquire the same knowledge from the same information, it can only result in sufficient similarity for understanding to take place (alignment). Secondly, a teacher's knowledge becomes the learner's information, knowledge resulting only when it is interpreted to give it new meaning. This may explain why "A" level graduates first need to transfer the information that they have "learnt" into knowledge by gaining experience, before they become useful to the systems they serve. There is a difference in the way that knowledge and skills are acquired. In the former, an internal transformation of information takes place, whilst the latter is acquired by repetition (conditioning). In other words, one may be skilful without having knowledge and one may know without having skills (*"He who can does. He who cannot teaches!"* - George Bernard Shaw (Cohen and Cohen, 1960)).

Learning: Altering Knowledge

Learning, and the ability to adapt, has a survival advantage. Companies and governments who have not learnt to adapt or have adapted too slowly go out of business (Ackoff, 1981). Adaptation and learning are also fundamental to systems methodologies (Churchman, 1979; Flood and Jackson, 1991). The process of learning takes place within a distinct sequence of events, and for the purpose of this book Kolb's (1984) system will be used. It is designed from a comprehensive and inclusive foundation, in other words, it satisfies the parameter of a broad view that is compatible with systems thinking.

Much of the process of learning has to do with altering knowledge, of which our mind maps are an important part.

Diagram 10: Kolb's Learning Cycle

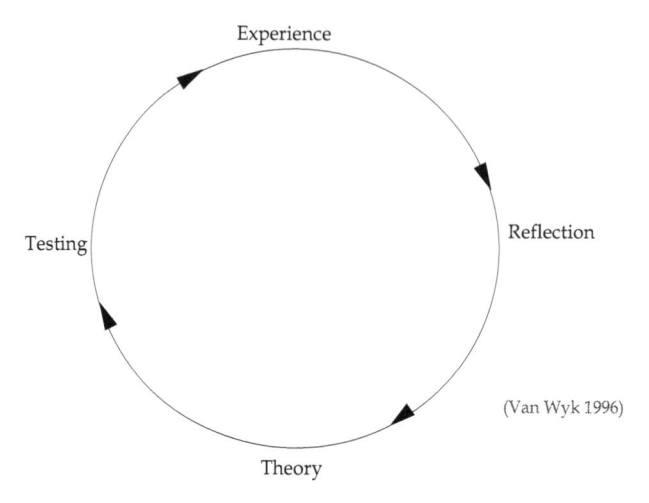

```
          Experience
              |
    Testing      Reflection
              |
           Theory
```

(Van Wyk 1996)

Kolb's learning cycle, in common with other learning cycles has four stages (**diagram 10**).

i. There is an *experience*.
ii. This is followed by *reflection* upon the experience. During this phase the experience is integrated with current knowledge. Further knowledge is gained by a process of inquiry, during which more information is collected in order to enable the reflective phase to be as complete as possible.
iii. *Generalization*. New actions are planned and a theory is formed (decision-making).
iv. Testing the hypothesis (*implementation*). This is followed by an experience of the result and the cycle is therefore completed and restarted by observing the outcome.

Kolb made the following important contributions to our understanding of the learning process.

- Learning is part of *experience*.
- Learning is based upon a process of *feedback* (it is a circular process).
- Learning is *purposeful* (the pragmatist position).

- Learning takes place as a result of *interaction* with the environment (a systems concept).
- All learning systems are essentially *similar*.

Kolb's philosophy of learning is based upon the action research of Kurt Lewin (1890 - 1940), John Dewey's (1859 - 1952) model of learning and Jean Piaget's model of cognitive development. It was also influenced by the work of the Brazilian educator Paulo Freire (born 1921), the social theorist Ivan Illich (born 1926) and the philosopher Stephen Pepper.

Lewin's work emphasizes the immediacy of experience to validate and test abstract concepts, and secondly is based upon feedback processes (a cycle). The latter provides a basis for a continuous process of goal-directed action and the evaluation of the consequences of the action. Dewey contributes towards a philosophical base for Kolb's concept of learning by introducing the idea of purpose (the pragmatist position). The concept of personal observation based upon experience of the environment is Piaget's contribution.

Kolb makes the important observation that not only these models of learning, but also others are remarkably similar. He infers that learning by experience:

- Is best conceived as a *process* and not in terms of outcomes;
- Is a *continuous* process based upon experience;
- Requires the *resolution of conflicts* between dialectically opposed modes of adaptation to the world (polarity) (a position similar to that of Hegel and later Singer);
- Is a *holistic* process of adaptation to the world (i.e. systemic); and
- Involves *transactions* between people and their environment.

Ideas are not fixed, but form and re-form through experience. Learning is therefore a process by which ideas are continuously changed. Knowledge is continuously formed from and tested in the experiences of the learner. The implication of this is not only that new ideas are introduced, but old ideas have to be modified or disposed of as well. Resistance occurs when new ideas are in conflict with or inconsistent with old ideas. The learning process can be facilitated when the beliefs and theories (mind maps) of learners are examined and tested before they are confronted with new ideas. This is the principle of a learning system and can be achieved in practice for example by the use of scenarios[1] (De Geus, 1988).

---

[1]*Scenarios* represent alternative outcomes in uncertain environments. They can assist in changing assumptions about the world (Wack, 1985).

Ideas that are integrated into people's belief systems tend to become more stable than ones that are substitutes for earlier ones. The former is easily reverted to in future states of uncertainty. The process of learning therefore consists of a continuous challenging of current mind maps and their adjustment. This has an important implication for planning and change.

According to Ackoff and Emery (1972) the processes of perception, consciousness, and memory, are used to form a description (mind map) and explanation (conception) of a situation. From the description and explanation, a set of beliefs is formed that are organized into a model (worldview).

Mind Maps: Shared Knowledge

In 1956 Kenneth Boulding wrote *The Image* (1987). In this work he described the idea that through knowledge we form images of the world, and that these images largely govern our behavior (this is similar to Bowler's (1981) concept of mapping, Piaget's schemes, and is central to Vickers' appreciative system concept). The image is based upon what individuals *believe* to be true, and is altered by messages received from the environment. Our image of the world is not uniformly certain or clear and tends to resist change, particularly if messages that are received are contrary to our value systems. To overcome the resistance, a very strong message is required, and when it is overcome, the effect will often be to reorganize or realign the whole knowledge structure as in the Kuhnian paradigm shift. The image also implicitly or explicitly has an influence on everything that we think or do (Flood and Jackson, 1991).

Image of self

One of the important images of early development is the image of self, or personality[2]. This is a complex image and subject to continuous adjustment under influence of the environment. The image that other people have of you, can influence the image that you have of yourself, and therefore also the ways that you act. Vickers (1980) makes the important point that images of social roles are vital for the functioning of a community. For example, if policemen or judges do not practice the roles expected of them, the concept of law that a community has cannot be applied.

Later in this book, it will be shown that the image that the community has of physicians as professionals has an important effect on the functioning of the health care system as a whole.

---

[2]The distinctive character or qualities of a person (Allen, 1992)

Resistance to change

The balancing of opposing forces ensures system stability. Systems will resist any drift towards polarity and the stronger the stimulus away from the mean, the stronger the resistance against it will be (Bowler, 1981). Mind maps are no different in this respect. Messages that are in defiance of an existing image will often be ignored or discarded. The more different they are the more likely they are to be resisted.

The opposite is also true. An example is the parable of the boiled frog. It has been said that if you heat the water in a pot with a frog inside slowly, it will boil before the frog will try to escape. The difference between the message and the image is small enough to be accepted until it is too late. The boiling is the price to be paid for imperfection. Mistakes in human communication are made all the time and are usually not even noticed unless the difference in perception leads to a significant problem. This imperfection ensures the necessary robustness that prevents us from being swamped by an overload of information, however, by increasing efficiency it sacrifices accuracy

Perfection of image

Knowledge is incorporated into an image. However, we have no way of corroborating the truth or accuracy of the knowledge or the image[3]. This is the age-old problem of philosophy, namely what is knowledge, and how do we recognize that our knowledge is correct. In the absence of reasoning, we assume our observation, and therefore knowledge, to be accurate. This is a potential source of error that affects the way we build more complex images or fact nets, leading to the same weakness inherent to logistic systems of reasoning (such as the Lockean inquirer that will be introduced in chapter 5). In other words, a small initial error can lead to a large error in more complex images developed from them. This then argues for the examination of knowledge by reason, rather than by intuition.

Shared images

Our mind map of the world includes a belief that it is shared by others who are in effect part of this image. Images develop as a part of the culture or subculture within which they develop. The concept of public knowledge depends upon the basic similarities of the ideas amongst people.

---

[3]According to Bateson (1979), science can disprove or improve a hypothesis, but never prove one beyond any doubt. Popper (Faure and Venter, 1993) takes this one step further by postulating that knowledge advances by the modification of earlier knowledge and therefore the acquisition of knowledge is the discovery and elimination of errors. The problems of scientific knowledge (or image) is the same as that of personal knowledge, the difference is only in the system involved.

This idea is also underlying to current belief systems about group learning. The object of group learning is to make shared images and assumptions explicit. In this way images can be altered or manipulated to the advantage of the group, corporation, and so on (Senge, 1990; Senge et al., 1994). The most successful organizations in the future are likely to be those who exhibit group learning (De Geus, 1988), in other words where learning will take place throughout the organization (learning organizations). Most of the assumptions we hold are acquired from a pool of culturally acceptable assumptions. In the same way we have assumptions about organizations, how they function, and our roles in it. These assumptions are often incorrect and learning about the organization takes place when they are challenged and altered. When the assumptions of groups in the organization are challenged, there is a tendency for members of the group to develop a better understanding of the assumptions of other members. In this way an alignment of ideas takes place and shared images are formed. This is fundamental for the functioning of organizations that are functioning as social systems.

The process of group dialogue is a useful practical method for revealing the incoherence of our thoughts (Bohm quoted in Senge, 1990) and to explore complex issues from many points of view. The aim of dialogue is not to seek agreement but to form a richer grasp of complex issues. Group dialogue makes a larger pool of meaning accessible to the group, in other words when members pool their collective ideas, the IQ of the group as a whole can be increased.

When two or more individuals share an image of sufficient similarity they may start acting purposefully together to the benefit of both. Once this happens a simple social system has been created. The decision to interact depends on the individual's purpose. Although controversial, there is a view that individual need satisfaction as described by Maslow (1968) may play a significant role in individual purpose. This model is based upon a holistic view of man, and consists of a hierarchy, (although it may be more realistic to conceive it as a continuum) progressing from simple to complex needs. The underlying philosophy is therefore essentially systems orientated. Maslow identified the following needs that individuals seek to satisfy:

- *Basic* needs. These are the simple physical needs created by physiological processes such as hunger, thirst, and so on.
- *Safety* needs. These are the desire for security, stability, protection, freedom from fear and chaos, and needs for structure, order and lawfulness.
- Need for *belongingness and love*. These are the needs for friends, affective relationships and group belonging.

- Need for *esteem*. The desire for power, achievement, recognition, and so on. The need for belonging is more concerned with affection as opposed to the need for respect, the context of which is determined by the internal judgment of a person.
- The need for *self-actualization*. This is the need to realize one's own potential.

In a society, culture, or organization, there is a public image, the essential characteristics of which are shared by the individuals in the group. A large part of the activity of a society is concerned with the transmission and protection of its public images. These images are also handed down to new generations by what Boulding calls a transcript. As a result of this transcript the associated value system will tend to select those messages that conform to the tradition of the transcript. An important image acquired by society is the value image. Establishments such as education play an important role in instilling the value system of a society, the most important reinforcement being from the peer group. Successful images often become the most dangerous when they become institutionalized. It is in this way that both the scientific and medical communities have managed to isolate themselves from their surrounding communities. It will be shown that the images of illness, professionals and health care are shared images and that they contribute towards the problems in the health care system.

Fact Nets: Organized Knowledge[4]

All perceptions or conceptions of the world (images), presuppose a set of *assumptions* that are necessary for relating objects with each other. Without these assumptions, it would be impossible to distinguish anything at all. Additionally, conceptions and relations that are linked together, and that support each other are linked together constructing a network of knowledge or *fact nets*. In such nets, new knowledge actively grows by the addition to, and by the modification and transformation of pre-existing knowledge.

Complete theories may be constructed by linking together statements that can all be proven true. However, it will never be possible to prove with certainty that the assumptions that we base our theories upon are absolutely true, hence it is impossible to construct complete theories. On the other hand, it is possible to approach an ideal of completeness by indefinitely improving upon our theories. When information is added to theories, the latter become better articulated, uncovering hidden gaps and inconsistencies, and increasing knowledge about remote implications of current assumptions. Hence, a quest for comprehensiveness raises new questions that when researched, will add to the growth and development of the theory.

---

[4]De Vree (1994).

Inconsistencies in a theory destroy the structure and order of the argument, causing existing knowledge to degenerate into unrelated information and data (increasing entropy). Adding to knowledge by improving the consistency of a theory, on the other hand, orders unrelated data and information into logical contexts (negentropy), increasing order and stability. However, at the same time, order constrains the context in which data and information is associated and therefore the growth of knowledge. The resistance against creating disorder in knowledge systems as described by Thomas Kuhn's (1962) paradigm theory may be explained in this way. Scientific inquiry, by correcting errors in theories, destroys the knowledge that it has helped to order, in other words, assists in Kuhn's paradigm shifts. Thus, a process of equilibration that builds up and destroys knowledge at the same time is desirable to prevent stagnation and decay.

The efficiency with which we adapt to a changing environment depends on the amount of knowledge available for taking action. A lack of information negatively affects our ability to survive and increased knowledge positively.

Knowledge In Decision-making

Peter Reason (1990) published the findings of his study of human errors in the book *Human Error*. Of importance for the purpose of this study is the decision-making process that eventually may lead to error. In his opinion a framework for cognition based upon modern thinking and research includes the following.

- Human information processing takes place either consciously (attentional mode), or unconsciously (schematic mode), and these two modes of cognitive control interact closely.
- Two structural features of human cognition may be distinguished, working memory (attentional control mode) and the knowledge base (schematic control mode).

The attentional mode is slow, requires a large amount of effort, and therefore cannot be sustained for more than brief periods of time. Hence, people will tend to avoid analytical reasoning in spite of the fact that it is a powerful means for problem solving.

Bartlett (1886 - 1969)[5] proposed the important notion of schemata, defined as an active organization of past reactions, and experiences, which must always be supposed to be operating in any well-adapted organic response. He emphasized that schemata are:

---

[5]Bartlett continued the gestalt tradition referred to earlier in the text.

- Unconscious mental structures (see mind maps)
- Composed of old knowledge; and
- Long-term memory comprises active knowledge structures.

Hence schemata reconstruct rather than reproduce past experiences, and Bartlett's schemata in effect are the same as Piaget's schemes and Boulding's images.

Modern schema theory sees schemata as high-level knowledge structures that contain informational variables. If current inputs fail to match these variables, they take on default assignments that are composed of past knowledge of the world. This ensures the rapid handling of information by humans, but on the downside, the price to pay for speed is an inaccurate system that errs in the direction of the familiar and expected.

The classical approach to decision-making is based upon research in the 1950's and 1960's that was influenced by American economics. This assumed that people always know what they want, and that they will always select the best course of action for getting it. This Subjective Expected Utility Theory (SEU) assumes:

- That people have a clearly defined ability to indicate their preferences on a mathematical scale when confronted with a number of future outcomes.
- That people have a clear and complete understanding of the possible strategies available to them.
- That they are able collectively to determine consistently the probable outcomes for each strategy.
- That they are able to select the strategy most likely to optimize their wants.

The problem is that in real life, people do not work out detailed scenarios and detailed probable outcomes for each scenario when making decisions. They are likely to ignore seemingly obvious candidate outcomes and seem to be insensitive to the importance of the ignored scenarios. Decisions are not thought through properly and also vary markedly between people. Hence, by ignoring the importance of a comprehensive inquiry, decision-making suffers from the myopia of a worm's eye view of the problem space. Furthermore, both individual and group decision-making will settle for satisfactory rather than optimal solutions (satisficing behavior). The decision-making process is complicated by the fact that people, even highly intelligent ones, tend to make the same mistakes even when presented with relatively simple problems. Reasoning tends to be based on similarity matching rather than logic. In addition, Tversky and Kahneman (1981) showed that in judging the probability of uncertain outcomes, people use a limited number of heuristics of which two, representativeness (like causes like), and availability (things that readily spring to mind) are the most useful.

Table 5: Classifying primary error types according to the cognitive stages at which they occur

Cognitive Stage	Primary Error Type
Planning	Mistakes (Failure or lack of expertise)
Storage	Lapses
Execution	Slips

Reason, J. *Human Error*. Copyright 1990 © Cambridge University Press. Reproduced with permission

Reason (1990) classifies errors according to the sequence of events that take place when humans take some form of action (**table 5**). Planning as a cognitive process is defined as the process of identifying a goal and deciding upon the means to implement it. It is during this phase that mistakes[6] take place because of a lack of knowledge or incorrect knowledge, and it is this stage that is of interest to the process of inquiry for the purpose of our argument. This classification basically follows Rasmussen's skill-rule-knowledge framework of cognitive control (**diagram 11**). Depending on the familiarity with the environment and task, tasks will be performed on a skill-based (SB), rule-based (RB), or knowledge-based (KB) level.

SB activities are primarily used for dealing with routine non-problematic situations in a familiar environment. Such actions take place mostly on a subconscious level with regular progress checks through a feed forward control system. In other words, subconscious checks are made at regular intervals and implementation continues as long as these checks match. When there is a mismatch, we become conscious of a problem situation and an attempt is made to revise the situation by referring to the next level of problem solving, namely the RB level. Accordingly, a problem may be defined as a situation that requires a revision of a current program of action (Reason, 1990). The schematic mode of control only functions satisfactorily when the current state of the environment matches a previously encountered situation, since humans prefer to function as context-specific pattern recognizers rather than active problem solvers.

At the RB level, attempts are made to match the problem situation to previously encountered situations, and if such a match is found, an attempt is made to resolve the problem by using the old knowledge. If successful,

---

[6]Mistakes are deficiencies or failures in the judgmental and/or inferential processes involved in the selection of an objective, or in the specification of the means to achieve it, irrespective of whether or not the actions directed by this decision scheme run according to plan (Reason, 1990)

further progress towards the goal state continues on the SB level. If not, further attempts are made at finding recognizable patterns on the RB level, and only when repeated cycling through this level is unsuccessful, will attempts be made at the KB level. It is at the KB level that mistakes occur as a result of a lack of or incorrect knowledge.

Diagram 11: Problem solving

Reason, J. *Human Error*. Copyright 1990 © Cambridge University Press.
Reproduced with permission.

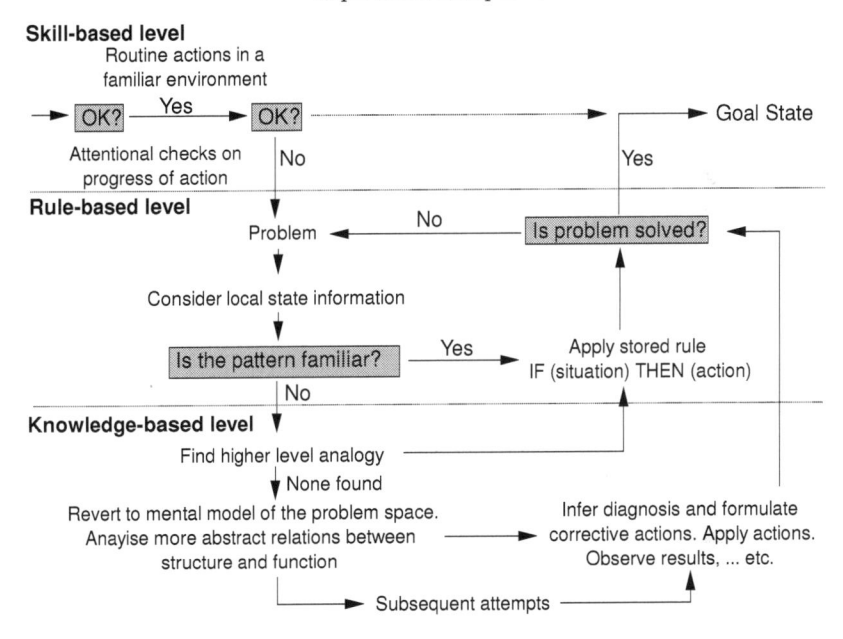

Skill-based level
Routine actions in a familiar environment

→ OK? —Yes→ OK? ···→ Goal State

Attentional checks on progress of action | No | Yes

Rule-based level ▼
Problem ←—No— Is problem solved? ←
▼
Consider local state information
▼
Is the pattern familiar? —Yes→ Apply stored rule
| No   IF (situation) THEN (action)

Knowledge-based level ▼
Find higher level analogy
▼ None found
Revert to mental model of the problem space.   Infer diagnosis and formulate
Anayise more abstract relations between   —→   corrective actions. Apply actions.
structure and function   Observe results, ... etc.
└——→ Subsequent attempts ——→

The quest of philosophy has been to improve our ability to reason logically, to increase our knowledge of the world in this way, and as a result to make better decisions. However, as Reason's work so elegantly shows, we are by nature too lazy to think, and when we are forced to do so, we do it in a sloppy way and with the minimum of effort that will ensure a reasonable outcome. There is an innate predictability in nature that allows the expediency of intuitive reasoning. This has been the problem of philosophy in general and even the systems approach; if knowledge based reasoning is mostly a hobby for those with the innate skill or interest to improve their ability to reason, how does one convince the disinterested majority to more regularly access their KB level of problem solving? It is possible to say that problem solving is a process that obeys the Second law of thermodynamics and hence will always tend towards greater entropy (disorder or incoherence). Furthermore, knowledge based reasoning requires energy in an effort to increase negentropy, therefore, the challenge is to encourage a system of knowledge and reasoning for the majority, in spite of the effort it requires.

We have seen earlier that reasoning may be analytical, such as in classical philosophy and science, or synthetic, such as in systems thinking. The thrust of the argument is that the latter, by virtue of its ability to inquire into problems in a comprehensive way, is the preferred method of the two. The next chapter is a summary of C West Churchman's systems philosophy, and more importantly, his contribution to our understanding of inquiry in a systemic way.

Chapter 5: Knowledge And Inquiry. C West Churchman's Systems Philosophy

Because of his writing style, C West Churchman's work is difficult to follow and understand. However, he made an important contribution towards our understanding of the process of rational inquiry. His work follows a developmental path spanning from 1948 to the present, and it is important to follow this path to understand his logic.

West Churchman was a pioneer of Operations Research (OR) and later the systems approach (Ulrich, 1988). He felt later in his life that the new discipline of Operations Research of which he was a founder had fallen into the trap of becoming just another mainstream discipline in establishment science, contrary to the ideal that he had of a multidisciplinary approach bridging many disciplines and approaches. As a result of this he felt himself more attracted to the systems approach, which approximates his belief in a holistic approach to inquiry more closely. He did warn however, that there are signs that the systems movement may follow a similar path to OR, using Systems Analysis as an example of an associated discipline that had taken on a narrow belief in measurement as central to its philosophy (Churchman, 1979)[1]. This statement is as valid today as when it was made originally. The search for rigid methodologies and areas of application for the systems approach amongst many researchers bears testimony to the fact that many people would like to see the discipline within a more mainstream environment. Churchman's work could be interpreted to mean that such an approach is not systemic and in fact anathema to the systems approach.

The crux of Churchman's work is that people as purposeful entities make decisions all the time, which can be made intuitively or via a coherent process of connected thinking, or logic. His interest was in how people make decisions and in finding ways of making decisions in a way that would reduce the risk of making mistakes.

In *Methods of Inquiry* (1950), Churchman and Ackoff gave an overview of the different Western philosophical traditions, and indicated the ways that each of them contributes to the process of inquiry. These traditions are still fundamental to most systems for inquiry used by the disciplines that adhere to the scientific tradition. They showed that each tradition on its own suffers from profound disadvantages, which makes it undesirable to use them as

---

[1] See also the imaginary debate between Herbert Simon and Churchman in Ulrich (1994b).

freestanding entities for manipulating knowledge. Of them all, the pragmatic tradition with its focus on goal satisfaction or purpose and method of controlled inquiry most closely approximates the ideal of a comprehensive system of inquiry. Although inquirers can never completely control the totality of the process of inquiry, they have a better chance of arriving at correct answers by using this rather than other methods of inquiry and intuition in particular.

In *The Design of Inquiring Systems* (1971) Churchman showed that each of the traditions described above could make a contribution towards the design of a more comprehensive, or inclusive system of inquiry. The Leibnizian inquirer contributes the concept of fact nets based on contingent truths, which is a fundamental point of departure for all inquiring systems. The Lockean inquirer adds consensus and measurement to fact nets, and the Kantian inquirer the concept of sweeping in opposing viewpoints of the problem situation. The Hegelian inquirer seeks to expand knowledge by adding different interpretations of the solution to the problem, which inter alia adds the value dimension to inquiry, and the Singerian inquirer contributes the concept of comprehensiveness based on Singer's producer-product model of causality. In other words, inquiry must aim include the totality of knowledge available in the problem environment that may contribute to an understanding of the object under study, an ideal that can never be attained but that can be approached forever. The book ends with thoughts about the importance of social inquiry, which is something that Churchman felt to be of great personal importance. He saw social inquiry as an important avenue towards securing improvement (betterment) of the human condition.

Churchman expanded on the concept of comprehensiveness in *The Systems Approach and Its Enemies* (1979). He pointed out that there are components of social inquiry, which cannot be quantified or understood by way of hard analysis, for which he coined the term "enemies". This is the intuitive way that people normally make decisions, and is an enemy because of the fact that it does not include different aspects of problem field. Ulrich (1994b) pointed out that ultimately a systems approach can only be rational if it is also able to reflect upon its own limitations, in other words by understanding the enemies[2] of the systems approach as a reflection of its own failure to be sufficiently comprehensive. This means that those who are critical of systems planning and comprehensiveness by virtue of the fact that they have to live the consequences of the plan are competent to be critical of design. Because they will be affected by the results of planning and design, the affected cannot be expected to voice their concerns in a rational way. Consequently, the rational approach to planning of a systems approach will always be in

---

[2]Ulrich interprets the term enemy to mean the irrational, which is in conflict with the systems approach, in other words the dialectic negation of the systems approach.

conflict with the subjective decision-making of the enemies. This opposition or tension represents a dialectic in terms of which improvement is only possible if the affected that are planned for are prepared to implement the plan, which implies that their concerns must be included in the planning process. To the affected, the planner's claim for comprehensiveness is an insult to their political, moral, religious, or aesthetic convictions, since politics, religion, morality, or aesthetics is what happens in the real world in which they live.

The following is a very brief interpretation of Churchman's work:

i. Inquiry can be either intuitive or logical, and the only feasible hope for making progress, successfully solving complex problems, and improving the human condition is by reason. However, reason by itself, contrary to popular belief is not perfect, and the shortcomings of logic must therefore be considered during any process of inquiry, something that can best be achieved by taking a broad enough view of the problem situation.
ii. No problem exists apart from the context of its preceding history. In the same way, inquiry is colored by the philosophical tradition of the Western cultural heritage. Various disciplines use aspects of the philosophical traditions during inquiry into and the process of acquiring knowledge. Knowledge of this tradition is therefore important to understand and design any inquiring system. It is also the basis more often than not for understanding the context of problem with which the designer is confronted.
iii. An important component of Churchman's design is the concept of comprehensiveness. Following the logic of a very subtle argument, each of the traditions make a specific contribution to, and are built into, the perspective of a more complete inquiring system as Churchman sees it. The outcome is a systems approach to inquiry and design. Churchman believes that the process of inquiry should be as wide-ranging as allowed by the scope of the inquiry. If the spectrum of inquiry is too narrow, important facts, questions, and insights will be missed, which may have a vital bearing on the eventual outcome. Because comprehensiveness is a fundamental tenet of the systems approach, this is the discipline best suited to satisfy this requirement.
iv. The problem and solution should not only be examined from the perspective of the process of inquiry followed, but should also include different other viewpoints to confirm the validity of the design and to ensure comprehensiveness. Only by including these viewpoints can comprehensiveness be ensured and consequently the requirements of a systems approach satisfied.
v. Finally, Churchman feels strongly that planning should only be implemented if it can be shown to contribute towards the betterment of

humankind. His insistence on an ethical approach is important, particularly in terms of this study.

Even if we are rigorous and exact in our inquiry, we must recognize that the method and conclusions are based on assumptions we make about the problem and life in general. These assumptions are fundamental to our ability to make life comprehensible and consequently for creating a framework from within which it becomes possible to function satisfactorily. Assumptions are also the seed for misunderstanding the problem, or the translation of the problem when communicated between people. In order to find truth, or a state approaching truth, we therefore have to consciously and rigorously analyze the assumptions on which our decisions are based. Reflection on the statements we make will often indicate the underlying subconscious structural and intellectual background from which they originated. If this background is incorrect or insufficient and made conscious, it can be altered to become a better reflection of the truth of a statement, or indicate in what way the statement should be altered to make it better. Reflection may lead to the realization that the network of assumptions that we function on often originates in the philosophical traditions mentioned earlier. According to Ulrich (1994b), the process of reflection and questioning can be realized by the use of the critical method of the Kantian inquirer.

The process of challenging and changing assumptions is based on a concept of perpetual cyclical inquiry, in other words a learning system. According to Churchman, inquiry in terms of the pragmatic tradition is a process continuously spiraling upward. Pragmatic planning is based upon the idea of ideals planning, which means that an end can never be achieved but can be approximated indefinitely through a process of continuous adjustment.

The value of Churchman's approach is the fact that it puts into position a framework within which we can ask questions (Ulrich, 1994a). In doing so, he does not attempt to answer questions to problems, and it is important to recognize that the framework is an interwoven mesh, the parts of which are difficult to separate into the tradition of a rigid framework.

The philosophical framework[3]

The Churchman philosophical framework is not necessarily a comprehensive or widely used classification, but it is sufficient for understanding the development of logic and thought in the Western tradition from its very beginnings. The thoughts and beliefs of philosophers are assigned to this

---

[3]All quotations in this part, directly or indirectly are from: C West Churchman and Russell L Ackoff, Methods of Inquiry. An Introduction to Philosophy and Scientific Method (1950), Educational Publishers Inc.: St Louis.

framework, although this may in some cases be an arbitrary assignment. But, the point of the framework is not to supply a scientific or scholarly analysis of the discipline of philosophy, but to create a framework for understanding the history and process of inquiry. To argue the nuances of the fine print serves no particular purpose towards the purpose of the framework. It is also not meant to be a comprehensive analysis of the history of philosophy, but rather to sketch the outlines of its development in a logical way. An understanding of this framework is vital to the understanding and application of the rest of Churchman's work. What follows is a summary of the more important aspects of the framework.

Rationalism

Rationalism is a belief in reason as the basis for certainty in knowledge (Allen, 1992). The assumption is that reason provides us with clear and distinct ideas and guides us to conclusions that we can draw from these ideas. A fundamental problem of the approach is how to identify clear and distinct ideas.

The rationalist idea culminated in Descartes' (1596 - 1650) comprehensive system, which signals the beginning of modern philosophy (Russell, 1993). He emphasized the importance of the reasoning ability within each individual with his famous *"cogito ergo sum"*, accordingly, only that which we can accept without doubt as being true is the truth. Descartes not only internalized the process of judging and verifying truth, but also regarded such truth as the starting point of all further knowledge. According to him, we discover truth by using rational intuition and whatever follows by way of rigorous reasoning can also be accepted as certain truth. The implication of this system of thought is that the roots, or beginning of truth is an absolute and pure truth, which is used to build or synthesize further truths or proofs. The foundational truths are derived by intuition and further truths arrived at by deductive reasoning, using the basic ideas as foundation.

One outcome of the Cartesian system is *reductionism*, i.e. to understand a problem break it down into its smallest parts and then analyze these individual parts to determine if they are absolutely true, after which the parts are reassembled again. This kind of system leads to the belief or assumption that the reassembled system will be optimal as far as function or truth is concerned. In other words, once the building blocks of the system are understood and optimized, the reassembled whole will be optimal and complete too. This assumption underlies most modern management and scientific methods implicitly or explicitly. It is also fundamental to the linear concept of causality.

Deduction

A theory or system of deduction is necessary to progress from an idea to a truth, of which two are in existence, namely the mathematical deductive system and formal logic. Philosophical deduction, or formal logic, usually associated with Aristotle (384 - 322 BC), is the alter ego of mathematical deduction. Both systems suffer from the same difficulty, namely what guarantee do we have that the initial truths grasped by intuition are absolutely true.

Spinoza attempted to address this problem by the law of contradiction which states it is impossible for a thing to be both A and non-A at the same time. Leibniz built on this law to formulate a modification of deduction as follows: start with a perfect definition of things, make no other assumptions except the law of contradiction, then derive all truths from these definitions and the law. He distinguishes between two kinds of truth, namely truth by reason or by fact. The first is necessary and the opposite impossible, and the second contingent and the opposite possible. In terms of this argument, the way things are defined is not important, as long as they are not contradictory. The fundamental problem, however, still exists, namely what guarantees the truth of the simple ideas? And in the end Leibniz has to resort to resolving the problem by using the ontological proof, which is not a proof of reality and the end result, therefore, necessarily is that rationalism cannot satisfactorily prove the objective truth of a statement. The logic implicit in Leibniz's approach results in the growth of interlinked facts, or *fact nets*. This concept will be explored further in the discussion of the design of inquiring systems.

The inability of rationalism to solve the problem of a guarantor for the truth of simple ideas resulted in the rationalist tradition in modern times being confined to metaphysics, where speculation and reason are the only methods used by the philosopher. In other words, the problem is sidestepped.

Empiricism

Empiricism is the school of belief that truth can be found by observation alone. Protagoras (500 - 411 BC) suggested that knowledge and perception is one and the same thing, from which it follows that the measure of what is true is within individual people. Following on him, Aristotle proposed that we are born with the ability to sense and develop a memory from what we sense and gain knowledge from repeated memories of what we experienced. A process is necessary to enable us to move from specific memories to general knowledge, which is called *induction*. However, the problem with induction also, is what guarantees do we have that the rule generated from our observations will always be absolutely true? In other words, even though we know that the sun comes up every morning, what guarantee is there that it will do so tomorrow? According to Aristotle the guarantor is *intuition*.

John Locke (1632 - 1704) established the foundation of empiricism, and according to him simple ideas reach the mind as a result of the working of perception, which precedes all rational processes. These sensations can then be expanded into forming more complex ideas by using abstraction, compounding or joining ideas, and relating or comparing ideas. When intuition acts on facts, generalizations are formed that are validated intuitively. The problem however is that if we have not observed certain events ourselves, we have to rely on evidence from other sources to verify that they are true, or that they are probably true. There is also the problem of whether intuition on its own is sufficient, and this guarantor problem leads to the notion in empiricism that there can be no certain knowledge in science, only *probable* truths. The outcome is statistical method of which the purpose is to measure the probability that an observation is true.

It is only logical that the real test for empiricism will come when we are dealing with abstract concepts that we cannot observe and therefore cannot sense, such as the existence of mind. Berkeley (1685 - 1753) suggested that the mind could only exist if it in turn is observed, and since the only over-observer is God, this brings us back to the ontological proof. In the final analysis then, empiricism finds itself in a position where knowledge is replaced by belief. All that we know with certainty are our impressions, and our beliefs are based upon intuition.

Criticism

As a result of the weaknesses of the rationalist and empiricist positions, Immanuel Kant (1724 - 1804) formulated the idea that both rational intuition and empirical observation are essential for inquiry and that neither can exist separately. He postulated that all knowledge begins with experience, but there are certain general assumptions that must be made in order to make observation possible.

The two most fundamental of these are the concepts of time and space. To recognize a train of events, we must observe the events to follow each other, which implies an underlying concept of time. Similarly, to observe an object it has to have a spatial relation within which it can be observed, which implies an underlying assumption of a concept of space. These assumptions before experience he called a priori, because they are necessary for understanding experience. Also, in order to understand the meaning of events in time, we have to assume that nature has an inherent regularity. It is important to note that Kant considered the tools necessary to measure experience, namely arithmetic and geometry, to be a priori as well.

Speculative method

This method is the modern expression of rationalism and proposes that at least some truths can be discovered independently of observation. Its application today is almost exclusively confined to the fields of metaphysics (ontology and epistemology), theology, and ethics. It is of more than passing interest to note that some of the more prominent concepts of modern sociology spring from this basis.

Hegel (1770 - 1831) can claim to be the thinker most responsible for the development of this method. He argued that to arrive at truth is not a deductive process by reduction, but instead a synthetic process, which he called the *dialectic method*. In terms of modern rationalism, the mind can grasp wholes or generalities on the basis of experience. These generalities are essential for truth and therefore prior to science. Metaphysical truth is therefore the result of creative acts in the mind.

Positivistic method

This represents the 19th Century extension of empiricism and stands in direct opposition to the speculative method, by combining elements of rationalism, empiricism and criticism, although in its final formulation it is mostly empirical. Logical analysis, as it became known, is an attempt to establish a scientific method based on purely empirical grounds and in the process it attempts to deny all deductive and speculative metaphysics.

Logical positivism

This school has its roots in Leibniz's logical analysis, which was developed further by thinkers such as Boole (1815 - 1864), Peirce (1839 - 1914) and Frege (1848 - 1925) and culminated in its modern form in the work of Bertrand Russell (1872 - 1970). The aim of logical positivism is to produce clear and precise formulations of logic and mathematics via symbolic language, which enables the analysis of formal system construction. In the Kantian sense, the world is meaningless without a guiding framework of interpretation, and for logical positivism meaning is possible by the analysis of language construction.

Sentences can be logically true or false (contradictions), or factually true or false, in addition to which there are emotive expressions without cognitive meaning, which are only important in the analysis of ethics. Science can be divided into formal science, about which analytic statements established by logic and mathematics can be made, and empirical science to which synthetic statements based upon fact apply. Logical positivism concerns itself mostly with the former by studying the form of language used to express statements. In other words, truth depends on how correctly the structure of the language was used to make the expression.

Pragmatism

Pragmatism represents an attempt to synthesize a theory incorporating the strengths of both rationalism and empiricism, but avoiding their weaknesses. It is based on the work of Peirce (1839 - 1914), James (1842 - 1909) and Schiller (1864 - 1937), and modern exponents of the theory are Dewey (1859 - 1952) and Singer, under whom Churchman studied.

In terms of the pragmatic approach to science:

i. The inquirer must have prior knowledge of some laws and facts, but these are uncertain and not a fixed starting point for inquiry. Questions of science cannot be answered with certainty, and in fact people accept propositions as true not because they are valid, but because they fulfill the criteria of the norms of a certain community. Therefore, truth depends on the purpose of the investigation.
ii. Science strives for error-free solutions, which is an ideal that can be approximated but never attained. The corollary to this is that for ideal truth error and risk has been reduced to zero.

The pragmatic approach holds that the effort to found science on the basis of observation or theory alone failed to provide an adequate theory of scientific method. If science cannot begin with truth, it can attempt to end with truth, and science can therefore be seen as an instrument and purposeful system for pursuing objectives. Both theory and observation are essential as instruments for inquiry, as opposed to beginnings of objective truth. The pragmatic conception holds that truth is whatever works in practice, in other words whatever contributes to fulfilling a purpose, and inquiry is therefore a process used for solving problems.

Inquirers have goals, or ends, but are in doubt as to how they should proceed. Inquiry therefore starts when individuals begin to interact with their environment, by formulating the problem situation clearly. This is followed by analyses to determine whether any observable facts about problem exist, and from these facts a hypothesis is formed about a possible solution. Observed facts must therefore not be seen as evidence, but rather as indicators of a possible solution to the problem. The hypothesis can then be tested and the result of the test observed, which leads to a revised hypothesis, or new suggestions, and the process is repeated until the problem is resolved, in other words the goal is achieved. The process of inquiry therefore results in purpose or goal fulfillment.

Whereas Peirce and Dewey argue that if there is common agreement amongst investigators a proposal is true, Singer argues that to define truth the purpose defined by inquiry must go beyond individuals or societies, or in other words must be more comprehensive and inclusive. This school is known as *non-relativistic pragmatism*, which is characterized by two general tenets, namely

i. All problems of science are interrelated (which implies a systems approach)
ii. Progress must be judged from an ethical point of view, in other words not from what should be done, but what *ought* to be done.

In terms of a pragmatic method of inquiry for a science of ideals as proposed by Singer:

i. No experiment is ever brand new, since new problems arise out of old solutions, hence to understand a problem its history must be understood. The ideal is to make use of as much past and present research and data as possible, and to introduce the maximum amount of information into inquiry with the minimum waste of time and effort. Due to the fact that it is no longer possible for one person to know everything about anything, the collective involvement of scientists is necessary. The time of the self-sufficient scientist is past and the challenge now is to assemble collective inquiry across scientific barriers (which argues for a meta-approach, such as the systems approach).
ii. The scientific model is the scheme used by the experimenter to understand the underlying process of his study, and the process of model construction is a continuously changing one.
iii. The conditions under which data will be pertinent to the study need to be clearly specified and to do that an idealized experimental model must be constructed otherwise the result is a collection of an unstructured mass of facts.
iv. The purpose of measurement is to predict outcomes, and prediction is about how we decide our possible relationship to objects in the future.
v. Scientific inquiry strives to state all the possible answers to a given question in any context as a hypothesis that can be tested, and pragmatically the number and kinds of hypotheses depend on the purpose of the investigation. Presuppositions are the common perceptions between hypotheses that are used as the background for testing. Therefore, stating the common ground is extremely important.
vi. Observations are recorded by way of measurements, and no set of measurements is ever error-free or complete. Statistical theory is therefore used to determine the degree of error quantitatively and used to minimize the risk of selecting the wrong hypothesis.

Statistical methods however also rely on assumptions that must be included in the methodology.
vii. The risk of an experiment is a function of the chance for, and significance of a mistake being made, which introduces the need for including values in the design of the experimental model. In this way the goals of the experiment are made explicit as well as those parts that the experimenter would be prepared to sacrifice if the original goal cannot be achieved. The negative impact of error on the environment, including the human part of it, can also be determined.
viii. The methodology of the experiment must be clearly set down, so that other experimenters are able to understand and duplicate it, which, according to Churchman is not an easy task since it demands considerable knowledge of how people respond to instructions. The ideal is to design and describe an experiment in such a way that it can be repeated by any number of experimenters that will all produce essentially the same results. The planning of and instructions for gathering information must include the number of observations necessary to draw meaningful conclusions, which depends on the risk one is prepared to take when a conclusion is formulated, since it depends on the seriousness of a mistake and the chance that it may occur.
ix. Experimenters must draw conclusions about the findings of their inquiries in order to select an appropriate hypothesis. The degree of confirmation depends on the prior information we are willing to accept, the number of errors in the observations, the design of the experiments, and the number of observations and method for analyzing data and drawing conclusions from it.
x. A perfect result to the experiment would be a hypothesis that is perfectly confirmed and that is certain to lead to the attainment of an intended goal. The pragmatist position recognizes that the ideal of an experiment in perfect isolation cannot be achieved, since the outcome is influenced by the actions and participation of the experimenter.

Summary

In terms of this discussion, the pragmatist approach is well suited for purposeful inquiry as a human activity. Churchman follows Singer's non-relativistic pragmatism and in a sense explored and developed Singer's ideas. Singer's approach to pragmatism adds the important concepts that all problems are interrelated, and that to make progress ethics must be included in inquiry. The pragmatic approach in some ways compliments the systems approach, since its essential characteristics are:

- Purposefulness.
- Cyclical inquiry.

- Ends can be approached infinitely, but never attained.
- Agreement.
- Every problem has a history.
- The concept of the single expert is no longer valid.
- Measurement is used for prediction and to minimize risk.
- No inquiry can take place in a value free environment.

Churchman's design of inquiring systems[4]

Design and inquiry

According to Churchman, we attempt to change our environment for our own purpose, and we do so by designing systems that enable us to achieve the purpose. Design is therefore goal seeking, or purposeful, and can be recognized when:

- Someone consciously tries to distinguish between different sets of behavioral patterns.
- Someone consciously tries to determine which behavioral pattern will be most suitable to achieve a specific goal.
- Someone tries to communicate this process to others so that they can achieve similar goals in the manner that the design predicted.
- The process followed to achieve a goal is recorded in a methodology so that it can be used again if a similar problem occurs in the future; and
- The methodology identifies the complete relevant system and all of its components.

Churchman defines inquiry as an activity that produces knowledge. Knowledge, in turn is conceived of as a collection of information, or an activity or potential. In the latter sense, knowledge is the ability of a person to do something correctly. To know therefore, one has to be able to learn and adjust. *'Nothing touches the true depth of the human spirit so much as the act of knowing'* (Churchman, 1971). The fundamental point is therefore that ultimately inquiring systems are learning systems (Ulrich, 1988) and it follows that the design of an inquiring system is important to the learning that will take place.

---

[4]All quotations in this part, directly or indirectly are from: C West Churchman, The Design of Inquiring Systems. Basic Concepts of Systems and Organisation (1971). Basic Books Inc.: New York.

To be successful, design must be transformed into action or another design, but the central problem remains, namely how do we know that the knowledge we use for the design is valid?

Whole systems and goal seeking

Systems are purposeful, because some of their properties are functional. Whether or not something is a system is a design choice by the designer, and Churchman makes the point that purposeful systems are enormously complex. For something to be identified as a system, it needs to fulfill the following criteria.

i. The system is *purposeful*.
ii. The system has a *function*.
iii. The system has a *client* whose interests are served - the better the system performs, the better the interests of the client are served. The client is therefore indirectly the standard of how well the system performs.
iv. The system has *purposeful parts* that contribute to the function of the system.
v. The system has an *environment* that affects the function of the system.
vi. There is a *decision maker* who can change the functioning of the components of the system and therefore indirectly the system itself.
vii. There is a *designer* whose conceptualization of the nature of the system is such that it can potentially influence the actions of the decision maker.
viii. The designer's intention is to *change* the system to maximize its value to the client.
ix. The system has a built in *guarantee* that the designer's intention can ultimately be realized.

The client, decision maker and designer are purposeful individuals who can produce alternative ways that will lead to desired goals. In other words, they have a number of possible futures in mind with a preference for some and to obtain this, they have a set of objectives, or goals. The designer has to imagine an environment in which clients can potentially achieve their goals within the limits of available resources, in other words constrained by the system's environment. This implies a trade-off of what clients are prepared to sacrifice in order to achieve their goal as near as possible. To be successful, the designer must have a value system aligned with or similar to the client's.

One of the critical problems for the designer is to identify client and decision maker correctly. The former is the person or entity, whose interest ought to be served by the system, but since the systems approach is incompatible with short or medium term goals it is necessary to have a client who understands the importance of long-term planning.

The decision maker controls the resources needed to change the system and therefore is a co-creator of the future, and its value system is not necessarily similar to that of the client or designer. Another co-producer of change is the environment, which is not under the control of the decision maker.

The designer, or planner's role is to attempt to guide decision makers into changing their value systems to a position compatible with that of the client. Agreement between client, decision maker and planner is important and fundamental to systems methodologies, but contributing to complexity is the fact that the client, decision maker and designer may all be the same person or institution.

Not all purposeful entities are systems, and the designer will therefore regard an entity as a system, only if:

- It is purposeful and has a function.
- It has purposeful parts, each with a function; and
- It is possible to conceptualize how changes in the performance of the parts will produce changes in the performance of the system.

Designers must have a theory about the system as well as of their own role so that they can form an understanding of how they can learn from the system and how they may influence it. The parts of a system cannot be separated in a design sense, but parts are identified in practice in order to obtain information about the effectiveness of the components of a system, including the setting of system boundaries, which is an arbitrary choice.

Finally, the design must include some form of guarantee that it can succeed otherwise there is no purpose in designing it, which can to some extent be done by designing in design stability.

A theory of knowledge

Central to most disciplines in science and also to many schools of philosophy, is the belief that the mind begins with simple things first and then builds this knowledge into a higher level of complexity. Secondly, the simple things that the mind begins with are considered to be inputs, either by sensory experience, or from innate knowledge. Knowledge is perceived as a given, but the problem as pointed out earlier is that we do not know if these inputs are an accurate point of departure. In terms of this argument, design can either begin with:

- Clear and distinct elementary inputs.
- Clear and distinct ideas that are not inputs.
- Unclear inputs; or
- Unclear material that is not an input.

The applicability of this refers to the Churchmanian philosophical framework discussed earlier. There is a subtle element of design in this discussion that builds itself into a comprehensive system of inquiry, which refers respectively to the following elements.

- Fact nets; the Leibnizian, or rationalistic system.
- Agreement; the Lockean, or empirical system.
- Representativeness; the Kantian, or speculative system.
- Dialectic; the Hegelian, or modern rationalistic system; and
- Progress; the Singerian, or pragmatic system.

The object of the discussion is a design base open to its beginnings and in control of all the material in its possession, and together with this, input should be understood in terms of whether control of the origin of the system's material lies in or outside it. The Leibnizian system accepts that choice is part of the system and is therefore fundamental to all subsequent design.

Fact nets

For Leibniz, design does not begin with clear and distinct truths. To begin with, the system must identify sentences and then apply fundamental laws of logic to determine which sentences are necessarily true, self-contradictory, or contingent (neither of the two). The Leibnizian processor only analyses the form of the sentences proposed to it. If a sentence follows logically from the definitions it is necessarily true. For the modern inquirer, all sentences are contingent.

The Leibnizian system provides a framework for creating a storehouse of knowledge in which knowledge is linked together in *fact nets* that gradually expand sets of contingent truths interlinked by appropriate relationships. The underlying principle is the idea that these fact nets will ultimately converge towards an absolute and ultimate truth.

It is widely used in modern science to form hypotheses and theories. Results that fit existing fact nets are more easily accepted than facts not conforming to current theory. The latter are often ignored, because to accept them could endanger the privileged theoretical laws at the base of fact nets.

For the Leibnizian processor, perception originates *within* the system. A candidate sentence forms when segments of perception are retrieved from memory and combined by means of imagination. The sentence is then processed through stored rules of logic and becomes a contingent truth if it is neither necessarily true, nor self-contradictory, and can be linked to other sentences in memory. Contingent truths therefore become linked together in fact nets, which grow in response to the continuing perception stream. Contingent truths at the bottom of the net become privileged, since they are implied by most other sentences in the net, therefore if they are falsified, the whole net collapses. The Leibnizian inquirer is therefore a model builder and contains all the elements that it will ever need internally, and it uses these to search the fact stream only for those sentences that form part of a coherent whole.

In terms of design, the system contributes two important concepts, namely the need for an a priori theory to begin inquiry, and the notion that all systems are fundamentally alike in the design of their components.

Agreement

The Leibnizian inquirer however leaves two design problems, namely what are the innate truths that fact nets begin with, and who guarantees that they are true? To avoid the possibility of beginning fact nets with fallacies created entirely by the human mind, the inquiring system therefore needs a way for identifying only those contingent truths that appear to be valid. The fundamental problem with the Leibnizian inquirer therefore is that it cannot identify irrelevant and discard false data.

Empiricism attempts to solve the dilemma from the position that items obtained by direct sensory input have a quality that by itself makes the item relevant and reliable. In other words, I trust what I observe. Observation is an obvious candidate for this role, but we know that the environment or our own imagination can influence our senses.

The ideal of the Lockean system is to identify the simplest observation that is fundamentally true and can serve as basis for identifying contingent truths. To do so, it creates a community of observers that has to agree about what they observe, hence the Lockean inquirer is an attempt to design a community of minds that agree about their response to external stimuli, or observation. However, there is not a simple way to design agreement, or even confirm that agreement exists when one suspects that there is agreement, since the Lockean system has no built in priori assumptions about the world to start from.

The Lockean inquirer not only can receive inputs, but it can also recognize the fact that it did so, and from this basis can act upon the information by labeling it. These inner processes or reflections can then be shared with other inquirers, and transformed into reliable sentences or simple statements of fact, if the whole community of inquirers agree to it.

Inquiry begins when an entity is observed. Basic properties are added to this observation to form simple ideas on which the inquirer then reflects internally, therefore, any idea in the Lockean system can always be logically traced back to its simplest elements. The information is only meaningful if it can be used for a purpose, and for this to happen, a number people who belong to the system must be in agreement about what was observed and the way it was constructed into a specific item. The design problem therefore becomes how to build in a measure of how the members of the system observe. Design will be successful when all the members of the community can agree that an observation is simple and are then able to generate true sentences from this basis.

Diagram 12: Lockean Agreement

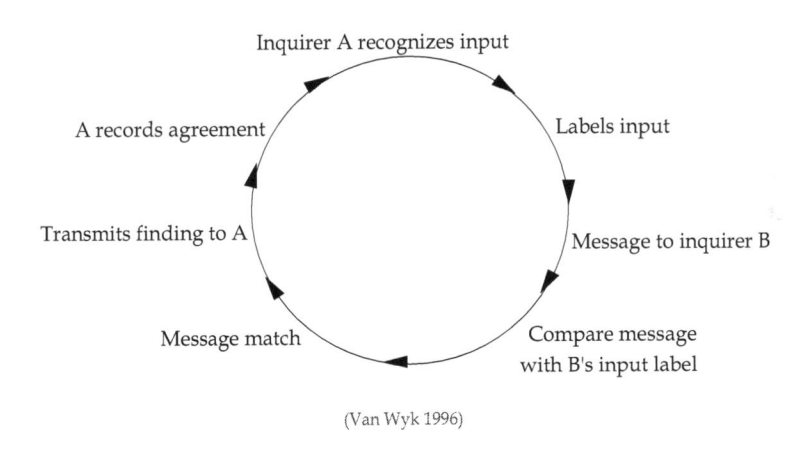

Inquirer A recognizes input
A records agreement
Labels input
Transmits finding to A
Message to inquirer B
Message match
Compare message with B's input label

(Van Wyk 1996)

Inquiry therefore also becomes inquiry into the community of inquirers, and the significance of the system is supported by the fact that other systems of similar design exist. This community of inquirers is necessary for verifying empirical truth, but not sufficient. There is only agreement if an overwhelming majority of members agree on the meaning of a simple observation. Agreement amongst inquirers should therefore actually lead to a deeper inquiry into the circumstances of agreement and not to a termination of the process, and agreement as the end point of inquiry may therefore be an indication of incorrect design.

Agreement is a circular process (**diagram 12**), and it is important to be aware of the fact that agreement is a human quality and part of a human activity system. Recognizing this creates a problem as far as the objectivity of design is concerned. The empirical tradition attempts to separate the inquirer from its environment and larger system in its design, however, if the one accepts that the inquirer is intimately related to its environment, the objectivity of empirical evidence is meaningful only in terms of the community's interaction with the system.

The goal of the inquirer is to create a large network of facts based on the empirical observations of the community. The community is designed in such a way as to stimulate a learning process during which an attempt is made to generalize experience via a process of induction. An important design question is whether generalizations in time influence the attitude of the community to the original elementary data.

The Lockean inquirer contributes the following to design.

- The problem of the guarantor of the Leibnizian system is replaced by the problem of a guarantor for the objectivity of inputs.
- The guarantor problem is solved by the design of a community along a structure that influences the way data inputs are recognized and the way generalizations are made from them.
- Induction does not solve the dilemma of a guarantor for the validity of the observations from which it starts?
- The objectivity of the inquirer is also determined by the larger system within which it functions and from which it cannot realistically isolate itself.

The Lockean inquirer addresses the Leibnizian problem of innate ideas and tries to solve the guarantor problem by way of the Lockean community. It leaves a new problem of design, namely how to design the community of inquires.

Representativeness

Any input of the empirical type must presuppose a formal structure that can be expressed in terms of a formal language. According to Kant, the sciences of geometry, arithmetic and kinematics are a priori built into the inquiring system in order to enable it to receive inputs. An immediate problem again is how are the assertions of these a priori sciences validated?

Kant asserts that if any of them were denied, the inquirer would be unable to receive any input at all. He implies that the inquiring system is capable of examining the methods by which it receives inputs and therefore of discovering the *presuppositions*, or assumptions underlying the method. This process of self-examination is important to validate the principles of its a priori sciences. The problem of validating is which of the apriori sciences is the correct one to select, which leaves the Kantian inquirer with two design questions, how does apriori structure influence selection, and how does the designer validate the apriori structure.

In many disciplines there is a strong tendency to separate the method of data collection from the method of creating theories. The two design sectors are kept apart with a minimum transfer of knowledge between them, and each sector is judged separately for its effectiveness. It follows that within an empirical inquirer the cause of unexplainable findings cannot be identified; one can only detect a problem in the process of inquiry.

This is not a problem in inquirers of the Leibnizian kind. Here, contradictions can be resolved by redefining the terms of the system, which makes it possible for the truths of one system to become the theories of another. By using this method, if the apriori structure is unable to explain events, a solution can be found by a redefinition of basic terms.

The way that information is presented has a strong influence on the success or failure of a solution. Also, not only does the problem solver search for a way to solve the problem, but also seeks to find the most economical (easy) method to do so. This creates a dilemma for optimal problem solving, because of a conflict between economy of method and the sparseness of information it implies, which leads to poverty of the problem solving process.

The richer Kantian design philosophy appears to address this problem. However, this design has the following critical design problems.

- Which are the simplest relevant inputs that are to be processed by the inquirer?
- How should the input be translated within the language of the model?
- How can it be determined whether the translated inputs provide a sufficient basis for translation?
- How does the designer know that a solution has been found?
- Is the design of a maximal apriori appropriate?

Dialectic

The aim of excellence in inquiry is *objectivity*. Any inquirer may test the validity of whether an inquiry is objective by testing the method of inquiry, which implies that someone (a master-observer) can observe the inquirer (Berkeley's dictum). For the Kantian inquirer, the inquirer should be able to see the same problem from different perspectives, and the Lockean inquirer confirms objectivity by way of agreement between members of the Lockean community. In terms of this argument, either an inquirer observes itself, or is observed by an independent observer. The problem is that independent inquirers can only observe what they see, in other words they have no insight into the inner workings of another inquirer.

The scientific tradition takes this argument to mean that the observer must be detached from the subject under observation. All forms of inquiry of this nature are therefore assumed to arise from the central set of operations, or sensations of the inquirer, bur these observations cannot be observed by another observer without losing the basis of objectivity. The inner core is able to attain direct knowledge, but the further you progress away from it, the more doubtful the abstractions of the inquiring system become, which eventually makes prediction in the system impossible.

According to Hegel, one mind observes another by a process of self-reflection, or self-consciousness. Objectivity therefore becomes a property of the observer of a subject, or a property of self-reflection, which is a necessary condition for objectivity but not sufficient. The restrictions of empirical inquiry may be removed if design is altered in such a way that sensations experienced by the inquirer can be self-observed as if a separate subject of observation in the same way that an independent inquirer would. In terms of this model, it becomes possible to observe and analyze the behavior of an individual inquirer or inquirers.

An alternative is to observe both observer and its outputs and also the interaction between inputs and outputs, or effect that the inquirer had on the interpretation of data. A response would be objective if the observer could observe both the observation and inner state of the inquirer and link every observation to a single inner state. This kind of system does not eliminate subjectivity since the dilemma is that the circumstances under which an object is represented cannot be captured in its essence.

The notion in science that the values of two or more inquirers cannot be compared comes from the subjectivist doctrine (Hume), and it also follows that subjective observations cannot be transmitted accurately between members of a community. This also implies that the value systems of different members of society cannot be compared apart from simply ordering preferences. The point therefore is that values cannot be measured in the same way as scientific measurements. Subjectivism also assumes that inquirers can observe what they observe accurately, which means that it is possible to distinguish between the personal knowledge of the observer, and the communal knowledge of the community of observers. To qualify to become communal knowledge, observations must be carefully controlled and observed and the inquirer must set down the method that was used in such a way that other inquirers are able to make exactly observation by following the process followed by the observer.

Observations can be classified as either mechanical, or purposeful. Mechanical observation either removes the observer from the subject under observation, or the subject is passive and the observer active. Observer and subject can therefore never be the same mind and by necessity are two opposites of a process. The former passes judgment on whether information is accurate, which is taken to be information independent of the experience of the subject, and an observation is confirmed as being objective if information from observing the subject conforms to reality. If information is factual (objective), it cannot change even if the inquiring mind changes.

Subjects are therefore dominated by fact, since they are not considered to be purposeful and have no choice about it. Hence, they are subjugated by information, or more accurately to the observer. The observer is deemed to be able to accurately determine the past states of the subject, a situation that cannot be changed by the latter. This mechanistic hypothesis is fundamental to many, if not most, aspects of existing intellectual and social life. Purposeful subjects, or people must accept the domination of observers and facts, because it comes from "experts" (physicists, doctors, politicians, and so on, a status achieved by peer recognition), they are a product of bureaucratic systems with built-in controls (accounting systems, educational systems, and so on, according to which those who participate in it accept the system), or it is of such a nature that they do not wish to disagree (weather predictions and so on).

In terms of the Hegelian inquirer, the master-observer is the collective mind of all individuals, and expertise therefore cannot be recognized in moral matters, accounts about souls, aid and philanthropy, and on the causes of war and poverty. Therefore, observers, or experts are able to inform about facts, but not values (this is a fundamental position of ideals planning referred to later on). Whether a purposeful subject benefits from delegating authority to the observer or expert or not is determined by the potential benefits of a policy; and the cost of implementing the policy. It is impossible to get an opinion without consulting the observer, and experts must be trusted, but they can sometimes be wrong, which constitutes the cost of a policy. In matters of ethics or values, experts disagree and therefore the cost of the policy is high.

Purposeful subjects agree to management by experts in those situations where the benefits of a policy outweigh the disadvantages, and in terms of this purposeful approach to knowledge, the facts provided by experts can be used to create the subject's own policy.

A purposeful inquiry begins by creating a worldview (weltanschauung). In terms of the teleological theory of information derives its validity from the worldview within which it is embedded, therefore, master-observers can only attain objective information if they select the correct worldview. Hegel substitutes the master-observer by the dialectical method, which starts by collecting information over as broad a spectrum as possible, which is then used to formulate a thesis. Data in defense of the thesis is interpreted in terms of a supporting worldview, or put differently reality is looked at in such a way that the data can be used to support the thesis. In the Hegelian inquirer the observer acts in opposition to the subject and proposes an antithesis based on observation of the subject. The antithesis is developed using the same data and worldview of the thesis, and out of the thesis and antithesis a new worldview, the synthesis, is developed. The act of forming a higher argument creates the conviction that this view is true. The cycle of argument and counter-argument will conceivably eventually eradicate all doubt, and the fact that the problem was examined from every conceivable angle ensures that it was observed objectively.

The problem of the Hegelian system is that mere analysis by thesis-antithesis does not guarantee that inquiry will be broad enough. It is also a system given to leisurely inquiry unconstrained by time and cost. Also, the thesis is only one viewpoint selected from a large number of options, and the question is therefore how it came to arise in the first instance.

The Lockean system then starts with fundamental data constructed into a story, the Kantian system tells the same story beginning from different viewpoints, and the Hegelian system tells two different stories using the same information.

Progress

Singer chose as his starting point the science of measurement or *metrology*. This means the steps that must be performed in order to make measurements and the way that these measurements are verified as accurate readings of some aspect of reality. Measurement is important for making comparisons between alternative options that may result in achieving a desired objective.

To measure, a unit and standard of measurement must be selected - the *unit* of measurement is an arbitrary choice, but the *standard* is not. In addition, a measuring system needs a rule-generating system to describe the methodology of measurement, someone to manufacture a measuring device, an observer that can follow the method and record its findings, and a second observer to verify the findings of the first observer, assuming that the first and second observers have the same measuring system. A measuring system is therefore based on a Lockean inquirer, or agreement, which depends strongly on the principle of a standard, namely a set of operations that will resolve any disagreement within the community of observers.

An important question is how do you measure the performance of the measuring system? In a length measuring system the important factor is to be able to replicate measurements, in other words repeated readings should be in agreement. If they are not, then the system does not accurately describe reality. On the other hand, readings that are in agreement do not necessarily imply that the system is working properly. The reasons for this may be that:

   i.   The measured object and measuring device remains unchanged over a period of time
   ii. The object fluctuates while the measuring device remains the same
   iii. The object remains the same, but the measuring device fluctuates; or
   iv. Both object and measuring device fluctuate.

This dilemma may be overcome by creating a Hegelian master-observer, since one would expect that in cases ii and iii a competent observer would be able to identify inconsistent readings when making independent observations. Competence, inconsistency and independence are judgments the master-observer must make, who must also determine whether the methodology was followed accurately and whether the observer's responses influenced observations.

If a hypothesis is tested and the readings confirm the theory, no amount of additional testing will decide whether another hypothesis based on the same data is false. Therefore, according to Singer, when all readings agree the system must shift to a higher level of refinement of the data, and this rule applies until a level is reached where not all readings agree. By applying this rule, the inquiring system commits itself to the assumption that every meaningful description of natural objects can be partitioned. This assumption is usually expressed as mathematical quantification, which assumes that nature can be reduced to a set of descriptions that cannot be partitioned any further. The Singerian system therefore applies measurement until the system reaches a level of refinement of its readings where not all readings agree.

A problem of disagreement about observations is to decide which of the four cases of relationship mentioned earlier is the cause of disagreement, i.e. an analysis of variation and whether variation or disagreement is significant or not. Hence, in the Lockean community disagreements are created to attain a higher level of agreement. The partitioning rule in the end states that if two contrary hypotheses are both consistent with a set of adjusted readings at a certain specified level of refinement, then there exists some higher level of measurement where one or both will fail to be consistent. This however does not take into account the resilience of general hypotheses about the natural world, or the strong relationship between hypotheses and readings. If a hypothesis is considered to be inconsistent with a set of readings, one of the following strategies may be followed, revise the hypothesis, revise the procedure for adjusting readings, or tolerate the inconsistency until more information becomes available.

Churchman calls a subtle and difficult design problem of the Singerian inquirer Kant's problem, which refers to the revision of the a priori, or underlying worldview. The decision to review depends on the purpose and measure of performance of the system. The Leibnizian system allows competition amongst worldviews, which means that revision depends on the relative weight of competing views. The Lockean system depends on a community of reasonable people who agree that a revision is necessary. Kant's position is that the community itself shares a common apriori mode for shaping and interpreting data, therefore, the question is whether the data can be shaped appropriately. And finally, the Hegelian system requires the creation of a counter-worldview once there is agreement, but it gives no indication of whether it will serve any purpose.

The philosophical tool of symbolic logic reveals the design features of proof but not discovery, in other words, *how* problems are to be solved rather than *which* problems ought to be solved. According to Singer, the attempt to reconstruct an inquiring system by logic alone is wrong since it does not expand the scope of inquiry, and the question then is what is the totality of the scope of inquiry?

In the Singerian system authority and control does not have to be included as a necessary part of design. These components incorrectly assume there is an authority or leadership in the inquiring system that can be referred to when in doubt. Control implies that there is a component present in the system that can observe and make corrections to it. In the Singerian system control and authority does not occupy a specific position in the system, in other words the system is controlled but has no controller, which therefore implies that the Singerian inquirer must include the total scope of inquiry in order to be able to authorize and control its procedures.

To revise readings the Singerian system uses a sweeping-in process. This means that inquiry begins with traditional logic and that further dimensions are added from other sciences, narratives, and viewpoints, while taking note of the dimensions of each additional viewpoint. The sweeping-in process therefore serves to overcome inconsistent readings, which in effect is another way of building a Leibnizian fact net.

A fundamental aspect of the Singerian inquirer is the fact that it is an endless process, because of the fact that the system is fundamentally an extension of the Hegelian system. In other words, when data and hypothesis are compatible, it is time to formulate an antithesis by measuring the existing thesis against a different standard, or viewpoint. The implication of the dialectical method is that two opposing processes are at work in the inquiring system all the time, or two sides of a coin are present, so to speak. The object of the Singerian system, opposite to the Lockean system, is not to resolve disputes by agreement, but to continuously stimulate debate about differences of opinion. It is therefore a purposeful system with an ethical base, and in terms of the earlier conditions mentioned for being identified as a purposeful system:

i. Its purpose is to generate knowledge for selecting the right means for achieving desired ends.
ii. The measure of its performance is its contribution towards the level of scientific and educational excellence of a society.
iii. The client is all mankind.
iv. The components are all available disciplines.
v. The environment is the total social system, since Singer's theory of value is based on assessing man's ability for attaining wants and not merely an assessment of goals.
vi. The decision makers are the heroes or people inspired to instigate change.
vii. and viii. The designers *ought* to be everyone and progress can be measured by the degree to which the designer, client, and decision maker are the same entity; and
ix. The guarantor is the betterment of mankind.

Finally, it would appear as if Singer's process of heroic change is in a dialectic opposition to progress, or the mechanisms of the production-science-co-operation trilogy of the 19th and 20th Centuries. The latter's aim is a world of enlightenment in which individuals are empowered to live out their lives according to their own individual wishes, whereas heroism is an effort to contribute towards the betterment of all of mankind. By insisting on an exclusive one-dimensional empirical approach, science failed in its effort to better society and progress can therefore be criticized for not delivering on its promise for a better life for every individual. The question is, can this be corrected by a more comprehensive approach to inquiry as suggested by the Singerian system and the systems approach?

Summary

To summarize, inquiry is the process by which we acquire knowledge, and according to Churchman a system for doing so can be designed by including a number of philosophical positions. Such a system of inquiry will have the following characteristics:

i. Knowledge begins with simple things that are sequentially synthesized into concepts of a higher complexity. In this way fact nets are constructed that are based on contingent truths.
ii. Contingent truths can be discovered by observation, however, there is no guarantee that observations are accurate and objective, and observations therefore must be verified by agreement between members of a community of observers.
iii. All forms of observation make some assumptions without which they have no meaning, and these assumptions can be discovered by self-examination.
iv. Objectivity can be confirmed by an external observer or internally by self-reflection. Observation can be either mechanical, where either observer or subject is passive, or purposeful. Mechanical systems are value-free and experts can discover knowledge about them, but purposeful systems are value-inclusive and therefore can have no experts. Values are true in terms of a pre-existing worldview, and such worldviews can be tested by a dialectic method that leads to a higher level of argument and therefore objectivity. In other words the dialectical method is useful for self-reflection.
v. Inquiry begins with logic and continues until there appears to a logical solution to the problem, or question. At this point other dimensions must be swept into the argument. The effect of this on inquiry is observed until there is agreement again, at which time more dimensions are swept in, and so on, therefore, inquiry has a timeless dimension. In terms of purposeful systems, when data appears to be consistent a dialectical process starts that will stimulate new debate. The purpose of this is to ensure that sufficient data is collected to guarantee the best possible decision and outcome. This has great importance for making value decisions, since mistakes in decision-making may be avoided by a sufficiently broad inquiry into the problem situation.

The Systems Approach

The systems view

Comprehensiveness

Design can either be approached simplistically when we feel the need to do something about a problem urgently (and embark on a road of possible disaster), or in a comprehensive way by taking a broad view, during which the consequences of any proposal are considered carefully by rational inquiry. The implication is that a comprehensive approach takes a long-term view and is therefore not suitable for finding immediate short-term solutions. One (and perhaps currently the only) such approach is a systems approach as basis for inquiry.

In terms of a systems approach, every problem exists as part of a larger environment and any change to the problem system will affect this environment, often in unforeseen and unwanted ways. The environmental fallacy of ignoring the environment during planning therefore states that it is more difficult and more important to identify the total environment of a problem than only its physical environment, but this is necessary to achieve a broader perspective of reality. This fallacy can be avoided by using a systems approach, in other words by taking a sufficiently broad view of the problem that satisfies the requirement for comprehensiveness of the Singerian inquirer.

Comprehensiveness, as stated before, means that a wide range of perspectives must be "swept in" during the pursuit of knowledge. Only once all possible perspectives have been swept in can we assume that what we know approaches truth or reality, even though complete truth is an ideal that can never be attained, but can be approximated indefinitely. Ulrich (1994b) explains that the ideal of comprehensiveness is to know all the facts pertaining to the problem before making a decision. Since this is impossible to do so, to be truly systemic one must acknowledge the fact that our perspective of the problem is and will remain incomplete. The Singerian position is that if we do not understand the problem sufficiently, we can sweep in more perspectives, or widen the inquiry until we do. The ideal is to be comprehensive, but pragmatically decisions eventually must be made based on an incomplete perspective of reality. We therefore must include into inquiry the knowledge that the planning and outcome may be distorted by this lack of comprehensiveness.

Worldview

Singer also proposed that all scientific inquiry is based upon the implicit or explicit underlying worldview (weltanschauung) of the inquirer, or scientist, and in effect what is tested in the classical laboratory are these assumptions. Scientists share such worldviews in the same discipline as a paradigm, and when Kuhn (1962) refers to the concept of a paradigm shift, it can be interpreted to mean that a collective worldview has changed, and an opposing worldview leading to the shift can be taken as an antithesis of a dialectical kind. In social systems the planner takes the traditional position of the scientist, and it is therefore the planner's own worldview that is being tested during the process of inquiry.

Measurement

The process of testing is subject to errors of observation and we can therefore only approximately estimate the truth of facts, which is why statistics has such an important role in the measurement and reporting of results. However, the experimenter is still faced with two possible errors, namely that we may reject some measurement that is actually correct (error of the first kind), or accept a measurement that is actually false (error of the second kind). When efforts are made to reduce the risk of an error of the first kind, the risk for an error of the second kind increases and vice versa. It is therefore critical to select the correct hypothesis to test to begin with, or ask the right question.

For Churchman science consists of two parts, namely traditional science driven by its own methodology and internal politics, and systems science, which is able to inquire into areas more relevant to the common good. Science has a theoretical component that is measurable, and a value component, which represents the ethical component of decisions made during the measuring process, and which for reasons identified before is usually ignored by traditional science. The dilemma with making precise measurements is that it works acceptably well in a closed "controlled" environment within which results are presumably predictable, such as in the typical laboratory. But the decision as to how to control the environment in itself is not only arbitrary, but also a value decision, although the traditional scientist may not be aware that this is the case. Furthermore, most scientific data is both theory and value laden and if either component is excluded, conclusions that are made cannot be comprehensive.

Most problems of management are vague, for which traditional measurement is ill suited, although scattergun measurement is a popular method in modern management science. This is also the conclusion that Checkland (1991) came to in his research. Hard system designs such as Systems Engineering, Systems Analysis and the RAND approach are suitable for well-structured problems, however, most problems where humans are involved are unstructured and the application of such methods is therefore ill suited for planning in these circumstances. In planning it is therefore more important to know *when* to measure than *how* to measure.

Ethics

Singer argued that ethics in the sense of appropriate goals for a system could also be swept into the decision-making process. This means that the important influence of individuals on systems must be recognized, and consideration given to the possibility that the objectives of the study may have unacceptable consequences.

Enemies

Finally, Churchman introduces an important concept into his approach to systems, namely the enemies of the systems approach. Much has been said and written about what he meant by this. It is this writer's interpretation that he meant the enemies to be the antithesis to the systems approach. The best way to see it would probably be similar to the Eastern concept of yin and yang, which is often misunderstood in the West to mean opposites. In reality it means opposites belonging together in order to make the existence of both possible, in other words without hate there can be no love and without the male, there can be no female, and so on. These opposites therefore represent polarities within the whole. In fact, without opposites there can be nothing at all (Watts, 1975; Capra, 1991).

The enemies then are the ways that decisions are usually made in real life by non-systems practitioners, and Churchman identifies these as politics, morality, religion and aesthetics. This is the illogical alter ego of the systems approach, which gives meaning to its existence and in the absence of which a systems approach would not be necessary. The implication is that no approach to planning can ever be complete without sweeping in, or considering these conflicting perspectives as well. In other words, in order to consider a problem in its widest possible sense, one must also consider how the enemies will attempt to solve the problem. Only once one has considered this can the approach to the problem have been truly systemic. It is of importance to know that the enemies often own or control the resources that are needed for change. They may therefore be decision makers that will determine whether a plan will be implemented or not, which makes it important to include their fears and wishes as part of planning, even though they may be illogical.

The enemies are defined as:

- *Politics*, or the power to influence and get things done and often aimed at enhancing personal power.
- *Religion* in the sense of the absolute, unconditional, unquestioned, dogmatic, and sometimes fanatical belief in the truth of something to the exclusion of all other viewpoints.
- *Morality*, or the choice between right and wrong made by excluding competing perspectives; and
- *Aesthetics*, or the intuitive choice between what is beautiful and ugly.

Lastly, we have to be aware that because the ideal of comprehensiveness is unattainable, planning is always based on an incomplete representation of reality. By using the systems approach we hope to make decisions more logically, but the enemies can also question the validity of this position. We therefore have to reflect on the fact that our view of completeness itself may be distorted (Ulrich, 1994b).

History of the problem

Churchman feels that a systems approach is incomplete if we do not examine the past history of a problem as well. We can only learn if we start off understanding the ideas and circumstances that contributed to and lead to the current problem situation as it is. The solution does not start with the problem, but with its history. Furthermore, the solution to the problem will carry within it the seeds for new and further problems, which will have to be solved in the future. Churchman sees the learning process as both the discovery of new things and the better understanding of old ones.

In this sense one also has to understand the history of the systems approach or the events that lead to its existence. We can conclude from the philosophical tradition that reason and observation are useful guides for contributing to a better society. According to Churchman (1979) *"intelligence, reflection, reason and observation, are the highest expression of living beings"*, which effectively reflects the aims of inquiry as a cycle, or learning system. The combination of reason and observation into a common system of inquiry is best reflected by the Kantian approach. Kant in essence postulated that what we observe largely depends upon our basic theory about the way that the world is constructed. For example, the historical belief that precise measurement of a system necessarily means that a description of a larger system will be precise too. This belief is value-free and has the potential for fatal errors.

The measurement approach is part of the worldview of modern management science, and it implies the use of various mathematical techniques to optimize, or minimize the outcomes of specific human interactions. The approach further expanded its application through the use of computers, which made long-term simulations of human interactions possible. The fundamental problem is that humans simply do not act according to mathematical laws. The enemies of the systems approach see to it that the realities of life cannot be conceptualized, measured, or approximated, i.e. social systems are essentially chaotic, or non-linear systems. Linear systems assume predictability over a period of time small initial errors will only result in a small error over time, but in non-linear systems, a small initial error is amplified logarithmically and the error over time may bear no relationship to the original position at all. It is therefore critically important in human systems to be aware of the fact that a theory is only valid in the first instance if the correct hypothesis is being tested.

Models and methods such as the systems approach are therefore also merely tools to find an approximate representation of reality, but based on the belief that they are better than other existing methods.

Logic

Truth

No statement or assumption can ever be accepted with complete certainty as being true or false. Churchman therefore follows Kant's definition of logic as the ways in which a statement can be *justified* as being true or false.

Worldview

Traditional logic as based on the Cartesian worldview assumes that comprehensiveness means that all the facts of nature can potentially be linked together in a comprehensive whole. The logic of nature therefore consists of dealing with the whole in terms of the way that these facts are interlinked with each other, or the parts. This is the fundamental foundation upon which the modern scientific laboratory is based. In other words, it is a place where we can search for and detect the facts of nature, which will eventually contribute to completing the puzzle of nature as a complete fact net. Many believe that the ultimate source of all knowledge is God and the assumption is therefore that it is eventually possible to have ultimate knowledge of God.

Control

In order to make traditional laboratory experiments possible, the environment in the laboratory must be controlled. Those factors in the environment that cannot be controlled are either included in the experiment, or removed from the experiment, which means that to science:

- A hypothesis is irrelevant if it cannot be tested in a classical (controlled) laboratory.
- The observer stands *outside* the experiment.
- Nature is logical and truthful, and any error in measurement is therefore observer-error, which can be eliminated by reviewing the results, or by repeating the experiment.

Although the classical laboratory is imperfect, it serves a purpose in examining nature. However, in the "laboratory" of society one deals with purposeful humans and during observation the number of variables introduced become too many and of too complex a nature to control. Social planning therefore cannot be separated from society, since humans cannot be isolated from the environment as in the laboratory, which introduces a multitude of variables that cannot be controlled and that may influence the outcome. Furthermore, the outcome also depends on the feedback of the people being studied and translating personal experience is fraught with difficulty of interpretation.

It is assumed in the classical laboratory that there are variables that the experimenter can control, and that if this goal cannot be attained that the design of the experiment is defective. In planning social systems, the variables are human and controlling them introduces an ethical or value question. If the planner or decision maker controls the action of the subjects, possible actions are eliminated, which impoverishes the possible outcomes of the experiment and also influences the validity of the results. Furthermore, a question mark hangs over whether it is ethical to control human subjects with or without their consent. An example would be the testing of drugs on human volunteers, although they are usually handsomely rewarded, the question is whether in spite of informed consent drug trials on humans is ethical. From the viewpoint of planners then, the source of the hypothesis is of vital importance and so is their own objectivity.

Methodology

This leads one to an important conclusion, namely that a methodology of problem solving should be designed in such a way that human bias is included as a central aspect. Such a system has:

i. A *decision maker* that controls means and consequently has the ability to change things in the environment. The result of change is either the realization of the decision maker's plans (ends), or the plan may not be realized and the outcome unintentional. Hence, a decision maker's actions may result in new problems, leading to new means, new ends, and so on, which is why planning is a never-ending process and learning cycle. Decision makers can change parts of the system under their control, but have to take decisions within the constraints created by the problem environment, which is not under their control. Hence, both the parts and environment can contribute to improvement of the situation, but only the former is under the control of the decision maker. This is complicated by the fact that the decision maker may not be only be a single person, but may be part of a complex interaction between various people.

ii. A *planner* that is the equivalent of the observer in the classical laboratory. According to Churchman, the role of the planner can be either:

    a) Problem solving, during which attempts are made to satisfy the goals (ends) of the decision maker for a fee (also called goals planning).

    b) Objectives planning, when there are constraints to the

solution such as that it should be legal, not damage the environment, and so on, but in spite of this it is possible for the investigation to go further than the goals specified by the decision maker.
c) Ideals planning when the ends of planning are determined by a general ethic rather than by the decision maker.

Diagram 13: Churchman's Learning Cycle

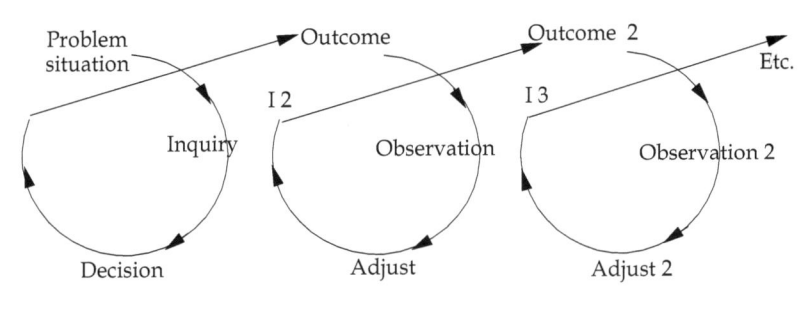

```
Problem         →Outcome         Outcome 2
situation                                         Etc.
              I 2              I 3
       Inquiry        Observation        Observation 2

    Decision         Adjust           Adjust 2
```

(Van Wyk 1996)

The systems approach to planning therefore involves adaptation, learning and correction (follow a learning cycle), rather than only being an approach for solving sequential problems such as classical science. It aims to base decisions on as complete an investigation as possible and then to observe the outcome, adjust the hypothesis, implement another change, observe the outcome, and so on, and must therefore be seen as a long-term cyclical process (see **diagram 13**).

The Churchmanian "methodology"

According to Churchman, people are the center of a planner's reality. In this sense, the application of the systems approach finds its full expression in the humanities. His planning system therefore assumes a purposeful human activity consisting of the following actors:

i. Clients
    a) Who have a purpose, and
    b) Who are the measure of whether the purpose was satisfactorily achieved.

ii. Decision makers
   a) Who control resources (system components or aspects of reality that can be changed), and
   b) Have a decision environment (aspects of reality that they cannot control).
iii. Planners
   a) Who have to know how to implement their plans, and
   b) What should guarantee that the plan would succeed
iii. Systems philosophy
   a) Which is used to identify the enemies of the systems approach, and
   b) To determine the significance of the whole effort, i.e. did it lead to human betterment?

Churchman never committed himself to a definitive methodology, since he felt that a framework is sufficient for gaining a better understanding of reality. There are therefore no fixed ideas and the process is always in a continuous state of flux. Since the process of understanding is not fixed, it is also not possible to commit to a rigid system of inquiry and planning. A rigid formal methodology has the advantage of precision, but lacks creativity. A more informal methodology lacks rigor, but has more creative possibilities. The latter is of more importance in unstructured environments than precision, which is the position taken by Checkland (1981) in his Soft Systems Methodology as well. A final and important point in Churchman's schema is a comparison between the realities of *"what is"* with the ethical question of *"what ought to be"*. Ulrich's (1994b) interpretation is that Churchman's questions are meant to reflect on the basic philosophy of planning rather than to serve as a rigid method for mapping reality.

Clients are people who cannot help themselves. If the starting point is who *ought* to be the client, value questions are introduced to begin with, which is why planners usually prefer to start with the simpler position of who is and what is the purpose of the client. Churchman (1979) defines purpose as future states of the world intended to occur by the decision maker that can be partially shaped by decision-making. Plans can be goals, which are executed in the short term, objectives whose implementation is over a longer term, or ideals, which can be approximated but never achieved fully.

In the case of goals, most aspects of the inquiry are given, that is both the client and decision maker as entities and the alternative options of the plan are clearly defined. This is the traditional hard systems approach, in other words there is a current situation and a desired goal, and the object of planning is inquiry into different possible ways of reaching this goal. In objectives planning, that which is given is placed within a larger environment and the outcome becomes that which is possible or realistic. In ideals planning, the environment is one in which all restraints have been removed. If this terminology is taken one step further, then the measure of performance for goals planning is the degree to which the goal or purpose has been achieved for the client. In ideals planning, the measurement includes the potential benefits and costs of the plan (in its widest sense) to the client and society. For the ideals planner, the idea is to improve the human condition (betterment) and it is therefore difficult to define a specific measure of performance. In the end, the most reasonable approach to measurement is a pragmatic one, which serves a different purpose for different people.

The *decision maker* not only decides on a specific course of action, but in the process also decides not to accept a number of other possible options. In goals planning a single person or body can be identified that will be presented with a menu of options from which one may be selected. The planner in this case is usually paid to study the consequences of implementing these options and to present a plan that will satisfy the client's goals. It appears to be important for humans to be able to confine the components of life within boundaries, which may serve the purpose of making what we observe more intelligible by putting it within Kant's space and time framework. However, the planner must never forget that the boundaries are arbitrary. They are also one of the central issues to be identified by both goals and objectives planners. For ideals planning, boundaries serve no particular purpose, since it is more concerned with the process of unfolding.

To the *planner*, the first question is who *ought* to plan, rather than who *is* planning. The fact is that we use our intellect in an attempt to improve our condition, however, only a few people have the training and ability to do so. On the other hand, the crucial skill of the planner is to bring together all the people whose expertise is needed to solve the problem (Ulrich, 1994b). Another problem is that expertise does not guarantee improvement, and the planner must therefore reflect on the possibility that sources of expertise are a possible source of deception.

Churchman (1979) defines Implementation as the transformation of an intellectually conceived plan into action, and this is the area where the planner and decision maker often come into conflict. In an organization there are often many co-producers that are necessary and have to interact constructively for a plan to come into being, and who operate in subtle and informal ways. They are often represented subconsciously in an organization's culture and can interfere with the implementation of plans. In objectives planning, the idea is to make what is subconscious conscious. I.e. make mind maps explicit. By doing so, the fact that some decisions and decision makers are manipulative because they change people's lives comes into the open. The planner must be careful not to be perceived as participating in manipulative processes, which can be addressed by participative planning.

Even then, it is an uncomfortable fact that many plans will never be implemented (Stacey, 1993). The goals planner experiences failed implementation as the inability or unwillingness of the decision maker to implement the plan, and the objectives planner considers the problem as part of the investigation into the problem. In other words, the reasons why the plan may be implemented become part of planning and the inquiry. Research by Churchman suggests that one of the reasons why plans are not implemented may be that people tend to be more comfortable when making communal decisions, rather having to make decisions individually. The explanation for this may be people's preferred cognitive styles (Kirton, 1989). The implication is that social groups are stability seeking and therefore gravitate towards an adaptive style, in other words communal decision-making (Van der Molen, 1989).

This raises an important issue which was never raised explicitly by Churchman, namely that of responsibility[5]. The traditional concept of responsibility is based upon the assumption that a person or persons control the resources and variables that produce a particular output. This is closely associated with machine thinking and the traditional linear concept of causality. In complex systems a non-linear environment operates in which the traditional causality model is meaningless. The magnitude of complexity in such a system is such that no individual can hope to control it. Therefore, responsibility in a complex non-linear system is meaningless.

Boundary

The boundaries of planning for the goals planner stop at the boundaries of the problem, and for the objectives planner at the boundaries of feasibility and responsibility, but for the ideals planner there are no limits. For the objectives planner, boundaries have to be set for the investigation of social systems, since otherwise the planning process never reaches the point of implementation. For ideals planning on the other hand, the major task of planning is to learn enough about the consequences of intervention to ensure "control" over the intended changes. Recommendations and implementation therefore become sources of learning. Churchman did not explore this very important theme any further and what follows is Ulrich's (1994b) interpretation.

Whenever a systems approach is used, strong assumptions are made about what belongs to the system under investigation and what is part of the

---

[5] *Responsible*: liable to be called to account; morally accountable for one's actions; capable of rational conduct (Allen, 1992).

environment. These judgments are boundary judgments. It is of vital importance to realize that these assumptions are judgments made by the planner and do not reflect reality. In many modern planning methodologies, attempts are made to define problems to suit the methodology, instead of the methodology being a tool for better understanding the problem. The former approach leads to problems with boundary judgments.

According to Ulrich, boundary judgments have to be made in terms of the boundary between the system under investigation and its environment, and within the selected system between those people who are potentially affected by the outcomes of planning and who have to live the consequences of planning, and those who are involved in the planning process through being able to contribute resources. This leads to two important questions namely firstly, what belongs to the problem and what to its environment, and secondly, how to draw the boundary between the involved and affected. Within this framework planning is influenced by:

- The client, who is the source of motivation (values)
- The decision maker, who is as the source of control (power); and
- The planner, who is as the source of expertise.

These three basic sources of influence constitute the *involved*. The *affected* are those who will have to live the consequences of the plan, but who do not directly influence the planning process. The affected and involved together constitute the social system that must be bounded.

Objectives versus ideals planning

A fundamental difference between objectives and ideals planning is that the former is under contract to a client, whereas the latter will invariably go beyond the intentions of the contractor. The objectives planner is morally and legally constrained in planning only by the ethical choice of whether to accept the conditions for working for the client or not. The ideals planner on the other hand strives for the betterment of mankind, who is therefore the client, and planning and boundaries therefore cannot be constrained in any way. According to Churchman, the ideals planner determines the ideals for planning for mankind based on its own theory about how values evolved in mankind, and the theory states inter alia that the conditions for the improvement of humankind could not be known, but in spite of this, all supposed conditions could be studied and questioned. The way that Ackoff implements Ideals Planning as a methodology therefore does not fully satisfy Churchman's criteria, since his approach is more focused on determining possible futures than on the explicitly bettering the lot of mankind.

For objectives planning, common sense is often used to avoid investigating options that are clearly undesirable (illegal, immoral, and so on). In ideals planning, all options have to be studied, including those that would normally be avoided by common sense, since otherwise the learning process may not be complete and the inquiry is not comprehensive. The implication of this is that it is logical that sometimes the implementation of the nonsensical solutions of the enemies of the systems approach may be preferable in order to improve mankind.

Participative planning

Although Churchman only mentions participation in passing in, it is fundamental to the concept of comprehensiveness and therefore to a systems approach to planning. The idea is that clients are enabled (empowered) to help themselves through participation in planning, and even more importantly, how to learn to do so continuously.

Fundamentally, in ideals planning of a system every stakeholder in affected by planning has a potentially important contribution to make, since in this kind of situation no one is an expert. The clients in such a system know better than experts what is needed and possible. Ulrich proposes that the planner as expert should only act to facilitate the process of inquiry. In addition, because participants participate in planning, they develop an understanding of the system in which to which they contribute and its interactions, the ways that decisions are made, and how their actions affect the system. Participation therefore leads to learning and personal development (Ackoff, 1981), and participants are enabled to build their own ideals and values into the design. Participation therefore goes a long way towards solving the implementation problem.

Ethics

A discussion on ethics[6] is fundamental to understanding Churchman's approach to ideals planning. His position is that modern works on Systems Analysis, planning, Operations Research, and so on all suffer from a lack of attention to ethical issues (Churchman, 1994). Ethics is (and has to be) part of the continuous dialectical process of discussion and debate, since in this way the Singerian system adds the value component to decision-making. The

---

[6] Definitions:
- *Ethic*: a set of *moral* principles.
- *Morals*: a) Concerned with the goodness or badness of human character or behaviour, or with the distinction between right and wrong, b) concerned with accepted rules and standards of human behaviour (Allen, 1992). Ethics can therefore be defined as: a set of principles to distinguish between right or wrong, or a set of principles for accepted rules and the standard of human behaviour.
- *Values*: one's principles, or *standards*; one's judgement of what is valuable or important in life.

ideal and reality are dialectical positions that are part of the same inquiry, and therefore both must be considered for a systems approach to be valid.

If a hypothetical question needs the input of an expert to solve it, it is a technical question. But if there is no precondition to the question, in other words it is a categorical one, anyone can decide on it, and it becomes a moral problem. Since, there are no experts on morality, those affected by decisions have the highest moral expertise to help decide categorical questions.

This raises question, namely that of the fundamental opposition between individual and social ethics. According to Carl Jung, individuals strive to individuate themselves, or to become integrated. To Churchman, Jung's theory implies that it is necessary for individual morality to be completed before social morality can exist, which in effect is a continuance of Kant's idea of ethics and is also fundamental to the religious philosophies of Christianity and Buddhism in particular (the bottom up approach). The antithesis to this is that if social ethics can extend far enough, it will provide a framework within which individual morality can develop, and the need for individuation on an individual basis will therefore disappear (the top down approach). Edgar Singer, Churchman's mentor, departs from this position, which means that collective morality enables individuals to individualize themselves more comprehensively within a moral system. Or in terms of Maslow's hierarchy of self, it becomes possible for individuals to realize their full potential in a system mature enough to create an environment that will enable them to do so.

For Singer, the good, or morality, must be found in purpose, in other words, goals or ends. In this sense ends are goals that can in principle be attained, and ideals[7] are unattainable but can be approximated indefinitely. It follows then that the answer to any meaningful question is an ideal and that reality is always an ideal. Since we are purposeful as human beings, we seek to attain goals and to do so we also want the power to realize these goals. The activities that improve the chances of reaching the goals, or empower the goal seeker are the means at the individual's disposal, knowledge, and co-operation with others.

Singer's position, then, in the end is that individual morality gathers it's meaning from within the context of service to mankind, in other words that service to other humans is the highest ideal, which Churchman calls heroism (hope). The implication of this state is a belief that we as humans *do* have the ability to improve our destiny. Churchman's position on heroism is perhaps one of the most difficult of his ideas to understand. Different authors have different interpretations of what Churchman means by this. Churchman

---

[7]*Ideal:* answering to one's highest conceptions (Allen, 1992).

explained in class[8] that he understands ethics to be the rational consideration, and morals the emotional judgment of what is right and wrong. Morals and ethics would therefore represent two aspects of a dialectical opposition, which can be synthesized into a concept of betterment.

Ulrich (1994a) on the other hand understands heroism to mean an evaluation of the *costs* of implementation of planning to the affected. Accordingly, the possible effect of the plan on the future of the affected must be swept into inquiry. This leaves the question of the measurement of improvement. Traditional ethics is inadequate as a measure of improvement of the whole system, because it relies on the moral and ethical judgment of individuals. Moral action is therefore identified in terms of individual action, and the ethical question must be understood in terms of the total system. To be systemically ethical, the "expert" (planner) must be knowledgeable in terms of the design, those who will be affected in the future (the unborn), and the harm that improvement may cause to the system as a whole. The challenge then becomes to assist the affected (client) into participating in making moral and ethical judgments. Since it is not possible to make binding moral judgments, the best we can to at present is to inquire into the deficiency of moral justification.

Ackoff (1981) elaborates on Singer's concept of aesthetics. According to him, the aesthetic function is to inspire us to create visions of improvement and give us the courage to pursue it. This means that we must always find new possibilities for progress and therefore we have to continuously create new visions for improvement. This explanation in many ways echoes Churchman's position of heroism.

Interpretation

Churchman's approach to planning can be summarized as follows:

i. The purpose of management is to plan the improvement of an existing situation.
ii. The process of planning is an ethical pursuit, and the purpose is therefore improvement for all mankind (betterment). Planning should consequently be based on the attainment of ideals and the ethics of whole systems.
iii. Planning is an intellectual (conscious) process by which we try to secure[9] improvement.
iv. Improvement is only possible if all of the conditions that will determine the quality of our decisions are considered

---

[8]JP Strümpfer, personal communication.
[9]To secure means that the improvement persists in the larger system over time. Churchman, quoted in Ulrich (1994a).

(comprehensiveness) (Ulrich, 1994a). To ensure comprehensiveness, one has to:
   a) Inquire into the whole system, in other words the approach must be systemic;
   b) Include the views and ideals of all those potentially affected by the plan; and
   c) Consider the possible cost of implementation of the design to those affected by but not part of it.
v. The process of inquiry must sweep in more and more aspects from the environment in order to be comprehensive.
vi. The starting point of inquiry is to identify the events that lead to the current situation, in other words determining the history of the problem. Different methods are used to inquire about problems and acquire the knowledge about it. These are:
   a) Fact nets: What are basic truths and how were they used to construct the identified theories and hypotheses?
   b) Empirical inquiry: How is agreement reached about the validity of the basic truths?
   c) Synthetic inquiry: What are the assumptions made about the sources of existing knowledge?
   e) Dialectic inquiry: What is the different view points about the knowledge arrived at by inquiry?
   f) Ethical inquiry: What is the value implication of the knowledge?
vii. We cannot design improvement without assuming some theory of the nature of the relevant system (Ulrich, 1994a). To be systemic, we must also reflect on the shortcomings and deception that this imposes on our planning effort.
viii. The crux of the approach is to view the problem from different perspectives in order to improve comprehensiveness. The problem is therefore observed in turn through the eyes of the affected (client), decision maker, and planner (expert). The problem is viewed both in terms of the current situation and the desired outcome.
ix. However, the ideal of total comprehensiveness cannot be attained. Because inquiry will always be incomplete, plans will have unforeseen results. We consequently have to be prepared to consider these possible outcomes and when they occur, must repeat the cycle of inquiry to enable further improvement. The approach is therefore based upon a perpetual cycle of inquiry or a learning system.
x. The inquiry also has to sweep in the perspectives of alternative approaches (its enemies) in order to be comprehensive.
xi. Lastly, the planner should inquire about the significance of the implementation of his plan. Management implies judgment about the needs and cost of implementation for the affected. An understanding of the consequences of our actions and omissions may be the only way to secure (guarantee) improvement that persists over time. We have to

ask ourselves whether the plan will contribute towards the betterment of mankind in an ethical way (Churchman, 1994).

Conclusion

In his writings, Churchman does not commit himself to a rigid methodology, but his writings in itself create a method that is immensely powerful and robust, since it can be molded to suit any particular situation. In this way it avoids the danger of rigidity that is typical of some systems methodologies and which inevitably leave them with deficiencies when they are not applied to suitable problems. By problems is meant the dilemmas pointed out in Flood and Jackson's (1991) grouping of systems methodologies, which for example suggests that there is no methodology currently available for addressing what they call complex-coercive problems. Churchman's work can be interpreted to mean that addressing the enemies does just that. The shortcoming is not in the methodology, but in the fact that certain aspects of human nature cannot be altered systemically or otherwise, and the search for a systems approach to do so is inevitably doomed to failure.

Churchman's work makes an important contribution to our understanding of the process of inquiry. In the second part of the text, it will be shown that the worldview of health care of patients and physicians contributes towards the inefficient functioning of the system. If this image can be altered, the needs, wants and expectations of patients and physicians may change, which in turn may improve the patient-physician interaction. Churchman's approach to inquiry is imminently suitable for testing the assumptions upon which all decision-making are based and in particular non-empirical decision-making On the other hand, it is also a powerful method for improving the quality of empirical decision-making based upon available medical knowledge. In the next section then, Churchman's concepts and methodology will be used for an inquiry into the assumptions upon which the prevailing worldview of health care, as well as medical knowledge is based.

Part 2: A Systems Approach To Health Care Planning

Introduction

The following definitions about health care will be operative throughout the rest of the text.

- Medicine is defined as: *The practice (professional work) of <u>diagnosis</u> and <u>treatment</u> and the <u>prevention</u> of disease.*
- Health care is defined as: *To look after a person's mental or physical condition* (Allen, 1992).

Diagram 14: The Health Care System

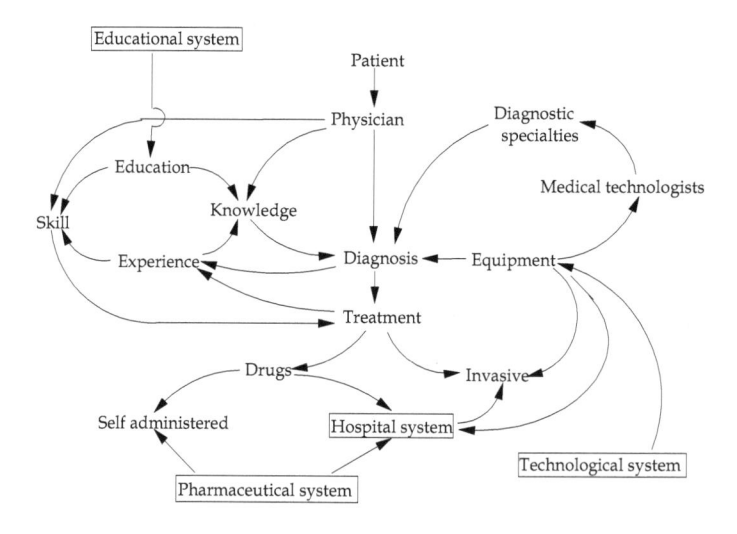

It would be fair to say that the traditional purpose of the health care system is to return ill members of the community (patients) to a state where they may be re-integrated into the community. In every community, there are members who agreed to obtain special knowledge and skills about illness and disease in order for them to assist patients back to a state of health. To practice medicine, they have to diagnose (identify) the problems that patients present with and treat them to the best of their knowledge and ability. Hence, the most fundamental component of a health care system is the patient-physician system, within which patients and physicians are linked to each other by the diagnostic system. It can be said that the patient-physician system is a system where patients consult a physician about a change in their physical or mental condition for the purpose of obtaining reassurance, or to have the change restored or altered to their satisfaction.

For physicians, to be able to diagnose and treat patients, the following is required (see **diagram 14**):

- Physicians use their knowledge to diagnose, and their skills to treat patients. Their knowledge is a product of their education, which in turn depends on the educational system, including the quality of teaching, continuous medical education (CME), the integration of research into fact nets, and so on.
- The process of diagnosis and treatment may lead to the acquisition of experience, which in turn may increase knowledge and skill.
- To diagnose, additional equipment may be necessary such as EKG machines, endoscopes, and so on. This requires a technological system that includes research, manufacturing, distribution, and the maintenance of equipment. Additionally, colleagues specialized in the diagnostic disciplines may perform diagnostic tests, which not only require special equipment, but also personnel trained in their use, such as medical technologists, radiographers, and so on. They in turn are also products of the educational system.
- A simplistic model of treatment divides this activity into the use of drugs, or invasive measures (surgery). Patients may self-medicate, or be given medication by health care workers in the hospital system. Medicines are supplied by a pharmaceutical system, which again includes activities such as research and development, manufacturing, and distribution. For invasive treatments, equipment such as scalpels, scissors, forceps, and so on are necessary, but more complex interventions may require lithotripters, laparoscopic instruments, anesthetic machines, and so on, which are all supplied by a technological system.

It becomes clearer from this model that a health care system that ensures an efficiently functioning patient-physician system is part of a complex web of sub-systems, and that the process of returning an ill patient back to the community depends on a number of highly complex interactions.

Health care systems all over the world are struggling to cope with the demands of increasingly complex interactions, as well as those of societal wants and needs. The most obvious symptom of this dysfunction is the exhaustion of a common resource, namely health care funding. A variety of organizations and disciplines are attempting to correct the problem, but they all suffer from the same disadvantage, namely a worm's eye view of the problem situation. It is proposed in this book that the solution lies in an approach that may convert thinking to a bird's eye view (concentrate on the whole), in other words a systems approach.

The next chapter is an evaluation of the mess experienced in medicine. This is followed by a historical analysis of the development of the health care system, at the end of which the reader should have a better understanding of the structure of the health care system. Chapter 8 examines health care process from the perspective of the patient-physician system as the most basic interaction of the system. Woven through all these chapters will by a perspective on the function and regulation of different components of the system. Chapter 9 is an analysis of methods used for addressing the health care problem and the reasons why they have been unsuccessful. In chapter 10 some of the assumptions about health care identified in earlier chapters are challenged and it is shown how this may contribute to an increase in the quality of thinking about health care systems and how the application of such thinking may contribute to their improvement. Systems thinking in general and the systems philosophy of C West Churchman in particular are fundamental to the discussion in part 2.

Chapter 6: The Problem Situation. Health Care Is A Mess

Russell Ackoff (1981) refers to a set of two or more interdependent problems that interact to constitute a problem system as a problematique. This is a French term that may be roughly translated as a mess. Messes are typically "wicked" because they are complex without any rational or even "slick" explanation, and they are often thrust upon us against our will (frequently as a result of some forgotten decision or intervention made at an earlier time)(Strümpfer, 1992). By definition, a mess is a system and to resolve it requires wholismic intervention, hence to gain understanding of the problem situation, it is necessary to identify in turn the system components process, structure, function, and stability, which are integral aspects of all systems. The insight that, in the manner of any kind of system, the nature of the problem is lost when the parts are separated from the whole is of vital importance.

An example of a mess that readily springs to mind is the worldwide troubles in health care. The problem situation expresses itself in numerous seemingly unrelated issues of which the most pressing is the inability to deliver affordable health care of an acceptable quality to the majority of mankind.

The problem situation

The modern version of the health care system is the product of a long history of interaction between communities and medical professionals (Knowles, 1973; Saward, 1973), and also an artifact of the Western scientific and philosophical tradition. The system in the first instance exists because of a need of social communities (Kuhn, 1962) for members who are prepared to tend to the health needs of individuals when they are no longer able to do so themselves. The health care system is therefore an inseparable part of society as a whole. Like many similar systems, the modern health care system is in conflict with its environment and also has to contend with a change of value systems away from the technological-scientific complex (De Wet, 1991). The result is that the profession is in a crisis with apparently no clear model or approach available that will ensure sustainable change.

Indications are that the Western style health care system failed to improve the health of people in many countries, particularly Third World and poorer countries. Even in the USA, a large number of the poor (37 million, or 14% of the population (Holtgrewe, 1993; Rothman, 1997)) do not have reasonable access to affordable health care. An important contribution to the failure is a cost crisis. The cost problem is a highly complex one. It is partially the result of worldwide economic realities and partly the result of spiraling medical costs that increased at a rate higher than the average inflation rate (Iglehart, 1991; Iglehart 1992a; Rothman, 1997).

Structure

The following are commonly considered to be the most important causes for the problem situation:

1. Budgetary constraints.
2. An over supply of physicians.
3. Unlimited patient demand.
4. High technology hospital based care.
5. Over servicing.
6. The ageing population.

Budgetary constraints

Most governments can no longer afford their contribution to health care (Fuchs, 1984). This is an economic problem to which the health care problem contributes, significantly in many countries. There are essentially four health care payment systems used in different countries of the world (Iglehart, 1991) and all of them, to differing degrees, struggle to contain cost.

A predominantly private sector model (USA, Switzerland, and South Africa)

In the USA health care spending increased by 1379% from 1967 to 1991 and was expected to be 3000% above 1967 levels by the year 2000 (Holtgrewe, 1993). In spite of this, life expectancy is lower and infant mortality rates higher than that of other First World countries, who by comparison spend less on health care. Additionally, an increasing number of patients are no longer able to afford increasingly expensive health care and are often left with no health care at all.

A national health system (NHS) model (UK, Sweden)

The health care cost crisis is not unique to countries with highly developed private systems. Britain's famous NHS has been suffering from the effects of cost constraints as well and efforts to restructure it into a more efficient system are well documented (Frankel, 1991; Glaser, 1993).

Social-insurance model (France, Germany, Netherlands)

This appears to be the model that has the best record at present (Iglehart, 1991). The fact that the system works is an indication that it is operating in a socially acceptable way to its members. It is a combination of government-mandated financing by both employers and employees, combined with the provision of private health care by physicians. Hospital expenditure is controlled and funds administered by non-profit organizations. In theory every German citizen has comprehensive medical cover with a free choice of physician. Most physicians are not allowed to administer hospital care and those that are registered to do so are salaried. An important reason why the German system works is German value systems. The German cultural preference is for reaching compromise before deadlock occurs. In other words, Germans are more likely to compromise and accept communal decisions than many other cultures, the implication being that their system will not necessarily work in other countries. Furthermore, the ability of competitors in this system to work together dulls the effect of the village commons type of cycle that is more noticeable in other countries.

Government health insurance model (Canada)

In Canada, the health care system is the nation's most popular publicly financed service (Iglehart, 1986). All of Canada's citizens receive care through their health schemes, which is the bulwark of the country's social programs. The problem is that Canada is facing a massive budget deficit, which means that support for health insurance plans has to be reduced. That is politically almost impossible to do since 80% of Canadians are happy with the plans as they are. Unlimited patient demand, no controls on provider volume, and an emphasis on in hospital care drive the health plans, a system that by comparison is very expensive. The Canadian provinces in 1986 paid 20 - 30% of their revenues over to health care. Government tried to resolve the problem by limiting the right of physicians to work in areas of their choice and by a reduction in physician salaries. As to be expected this led to an immediate confrontation with the medical profession.

Many governments nurtured for political gains unlimited access to health services without informing their constituents of the eventual cost attached to such benefits. The situation now exists where cost limits are probed and urgent solutions will have to be found to resolve the crisis.

Over supply of physicians

An important factor in rising health care costs is the number of physicians in the system (Wennberg quoted in Holtgrewe (1993)) and there is a worldwide over supply of physicians (Anonymous, 1991). The principle that the training of a larger number of physicians will lead to more competition and therefore cost containment (an economic model, based upon the mistaken assumption that health needs are finite) has had exactly the opposite effect (Glaser, 1993). It was projected that in the USA by the year 2000, there would be an oversupply of physicians in disciplines such as surgery, ophthalmology, gynecology, and so on, and equal demand in all remaining disciplines except psychiatry, in which there would be a shortage (Kaplan and Sadock, 1991). Every physician creates work to survive, some of which will be unnecessary or of dubious value (Holtgrewe, 1993). It is documented that there are twice as many surgeons per population in the USA as compared to England and Wales, and that they perform twice as much surgery (Bunker, 1970). There may be many reasons for this, but one is that the number of physicians determines the amount of work that will be performed (Illich, 1976; Wennberg, 1986).

In spite of the oversupply, there is a geographical maldistribution of physicians. Most physicians elect to work in more affluent metropolitan areas for obvious reasons (better income, better socio-economic environment, better education, and so forth) (Stimmel, 1992). For example, the patient-physician ratio in a developing country such as South Africa is within the recommended norm (Benade, 1992), but with 78% of physicians in metropolitan areas, they are severely maldistributed (Botha et al. 1986).

The belief that there is free market competition amongst physicians that may regulate the system is a fallacy. Competitors are eliminated constitutionally by regulating entrance to training and professional societies, hence preventing free access to the market. Laws that prevent physicians from practicing in countries other than their own does not protect the citizens of that country, it protects local physicians that are inept. Additionally, the inept are protected constitutionally by regulations preventing efficient and effective physicians from advertising their skills. The health care system can only respond to market forces if the constraints to free association are removed.

Unlimited patient demand

Unlimited patient demand (wants) as opposed to needs (needs *must* be satisfied but wants not) (Frankel, 1991; Samuelson, 1993). According to Hupkes (1992), the aim of economics is to find optimum ways for utilizing scarce resources, in order to maximize the satisfaction of needs. He divides needs and wants into those of the individual as opposed to that of the community. According to him, health care is not a commodity that can be bought or sold in the market place and will therefore not be influenced by the usual market forces. The problem is that the demand for health care is often a derived demand (be it primary or curative health services) determined by the suppliers. In other words, the health care system itself creates wants that will ensure its profitability (see also Illich (1976), and Rothman (1997)). The satisfaction of wants is often not to the patient's benefit (but usually cause no harm) and adds to the cost spiral. The result is the belief by both consumer and provider that health care is an infinite resource, an initial condition for a village commons type of situation. The economic reality is that no society can any longer support all of its social wants. Painful decisions will be necessary in future to establish priorities and needs, a scenario foreseen by Vickers (1984).

Most business management approaches to health care are based upon a needs-wants (supply-and-demand) model. The trouble is that the conditions that drive competition in the regular market place do not exist in health care (Teisberg and Porter, 1994). The reason was stated earlier, namely that health care is not a commodity and the rules for supply and demand are therefore not applicable to it. In other words, in system dynamics terms, there is no balancing loop. A commodity is usually conceived to be an article or raw material that can be bought and sold, in other words, a product as opposed to a service (Allen, 1992). Health care is a service and not a product and illness a need. Withholding or limiting a service of which the purpose is to satisfy a human need is ethically indefensible. The dilemma is with the satisfaction of wants.

High technology hospital based care

According to Holtgrewe (1993), before the 1930's Americans paid 80 - 90% of health care costs out of pocket. The introduction of hospital plans since then favored a system of hospital insurance rather than health insurance. This resulted in lucrative incomes for such institutions and consequently an emphasis on hospital based care. Additionally, they installed high technology facilities to attract physicians, and with them their patients, to ensure continuing profits (Marwick, 1992, Rothman, 1997). This created a market for high technology medical research. In the USA, the expenditure on medical research and development increased by 24000% from 1940 to 1970. The shift of emphasis had three unforeseen results.

a) A profitable business opportunity arose that was exploited vigorously.
b) Patient perception that the responsibility for cost containment shifted away from them.
c) An altered image of hospital based care as desirable for health.

Over servicing

There is evidence that the actions of physicians contribute to an increase in cost. Many health care systems are structured in such a way that physicians have an incentive to abuse the system. Studies show that a fee-for-service (FFS) remuneration system plays an important role in physician behavior (Anonymous, 1991; Broomberg, 1990; Broomberg and Price, 1990; Price and Broomberg, 1990). It also shows that the method of remuneration in a controlled health care environment influences decision-making (Hemenway et al. 1990; Hillman et al. 1989; Milstein et al. 1989).

Medical education is becoming extremely expensive. The ability to generate a high income to repay bursaries and study loans therefore becomes an imperative for newly qualified physicians in order to survive (Colborn, 1992; Stimmel, 1992). An early incentive is therefore created once qualified to abuse the system of payment.

There is a perception, with good reason, that physicians are amply remunerated and that this must be curtailed (Ragg, 1993). Furthermore, the perception is one of the causes for the high litigation rate in countries such as the USA (Claassen and Verschoor, 1992). Patients feel that physicians earn large amounts of money and therefore have to take more responsibility for their actions (Claassen and Verschoor, 1992; De Wet, 1991). Because highly complex interactions can only be partially controlled and physicians are liable to make mistakes, the result is litigation, high malpractice insurance fees, higher tariffs, and so on. In other words, a positive feed forward mechanism is created that reinforces the cost spiral.

Medical administrators often are in conflict with both patients and physicians. Their aim is to spend less than they receive in premiums. For physicians, it means that they are expected to assume costs for services already provided that neither administrator nor patient may want to pay for. That creates an incentive to recover losses in other ways (Teisberg and Porter, 1994).

The ageing population

It is a principle of most health care systems that the healthy young who are employed will cross-subsidize elderly retired people (Samuelson, 1993), who are more likely to suffer from chronic ill health (Glaser, 1993). People over 85 years of age have the highest per capita health costs and in some countries the elderly now account for more than a third of all health care expenditure (Anonymous, 1991; Faltermayer, 1994; Iglehart, 1992a). In theory, when the young retire, the next generation will in turn support them, and so on. However, most first world communities now have a zero or negative population growth rate. There are simply no longer enough younger people to subsidize the elderly. The unemployed are also cross-subsidized by the employed, and the ill by the well, hence the contribution towards health care is in effect a system for the transference of wealth (Holtgrewe, 1993).

Process

On the basis of the causes of the cost problem, the mess in health care appears deceptively simple. However, if these factors are linked by flow tracing (System Dynamics modeling) to demonstrate the ways in which they interact, the problem situation alters to express itself as a complex system with its attendant multiplicity of interactions and co-producers, complex causality, and time lags. Simplistic assumptions made about possible interventions based in isolation on the structural component of the mess become inappropriate when the process interactions are added to decision-making.

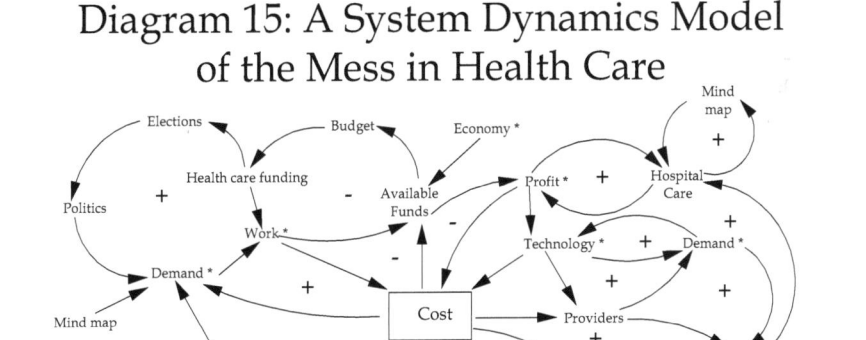

Diagram 15: A System Dynamics Model of the Mess in Health Care

(Van Wyk 1996)

The interactions illustrated in **diagram 15** are only the major ones. On closer inspection there are others that may also be relevant to the problem situation, such as the influence of the economic and educational systems. For the sake of readability, demand, economy, technology and profit have been inserted in more than one location in the diagram and are marked with an asterisk to denote this. This is an artificial separation and the correct interpretation is:

a) Demand for health care is created through election promises, improved technology, an ageing population, by service providers (creating work for themselves in order to increase profits), and as a result of the mind map of health. Increased demand leads to more work and hence increased cost, which feeds back to increase

125

demand. Increased profits lead to an increased demand for quality of care and feeds into the litigation loop. Demand loops are reinforcing loops.

b) The economy determines the amount of money available to governments for health care funding and education. It also determines employment opportunities and the income of economically active members of society who subsidize the elderly. Hence, it is part of the environment that cannot be controlled by health care decision-makers and constitutes a balancing loop.

c) Technology increases longevity by decreasing the death rate. It also contributes to patient demand for health care and attracts service providers to hospitals. These are all reinforcing loops.

d) Administrators, service providers, hospitals, and so forth profit from the system. They all compete for the same resource, namely health care funding. The profit motive is self-reinforcing, but the availability of the resource (funding) is balanced by the economy.

In terms of the system dynamics model, the structural components of the mess may be re-interpreted as follows.

a) Government budgets are constrained by the funds available to them. The biggest contribution to funding is made by taxing economically active citizens of a country. Part of the budget is for health care, and the delivery of health care in turn has an effect on available funds. Under normal circumstances this will be a balancing loop. In the Canadian example, available funds are limited as a result of economic factors in general, and therefore less funding becomes available for health care. The trouble is the effect of a second causality loop. Health care spending is popular and therefore has an effect on a political party's re-electability. Politics is about power (Ackoff, 1981) and promises are made during elections that lead to expectations from constituents. These are often demands for more and better health care, which leads to increased cost and therefore activates a reinforcing loop. In this case, the balance is disturbed by economic factors, which in turn affect the political system.

b) Service providers create work to increase profits, which affects cost. The belief that profits could be driven down through market forces by increasing the number of service providers, have had the opposite effect. This is a reinforcing loop.

c) Hospital based health care is profitable and therefore results in more of the same kind. Profits are used to invest in high technology equipment and techniques that may attract physicians and their patients, hence more work and more hospital care. High technology care also increases patient demand for alternative more expensive treatments and this in itself drives up cost. The latter is also affected by hospital profits. All these loops are reinforcing and jealously protected by vested interests.

d) A fee-for-service remuneration system maximizes profit, which in turn increases demand for more profits. Physicians affect the system in three other ways.
   i) Increasingly expensive medical education increases physician debt at qualification, which decreases their profitability and increases the need for high earnings. This is a reinforcing loop. Educational cost in terms of design is a separate problem that is influenced amongst other things by the educational system and economic factors.
   ii) Patients demand responsible actions from health care professionals because of the perception that they earn high incomes. This results in increased risk of litigation, higher malpractice insurance fees, decreased profit and therefore an incentive to recover profit in other ways. This is a reinforcing loop.
   iii) Lastly, medical administrators have an incentive for cost saving. Cost savings result in higher profitability for health care management and higher returns to investors. But savings are often perceived to be at the expense of physicians, resulting in higher consultation fees. In other words, an effort to decrease cost affect provider profit and an incentive is created to recover losses in other ways.

e) Animal populations are stabilized by opposing balancing loops for birth and death rate (Kauffman, 1980). The same applies to human systems. In terms of the health care system, the aged has increased health needs, which affects cost. The earnings of the young are the source of income for subsidizing the aged who no longer earns wages. The health care system contributes to longevity and at the same time intervenes with the birth rate through birth control. Factors that affect the ability of the young to earn, such as the economy, also indirectly affect the balance. This destabilization of a stable system has had an effect on another system, health care and the attending health care cost.

f) Cost is not only a symptom of the problem; at the same time it is also a balancing loop. Funding for health care is not finite and eventually the point will be reached where it is no longer possible to support profit at any level in the system. When this point is reached, some of the reinforcing causality loops will collapse and the whole system will become unstable. At the same time demands for wants will by necessity have to be replaced by needs and in all probability communal rather than individual needs.

Function and stability

Diagram 16: Balancing Funding

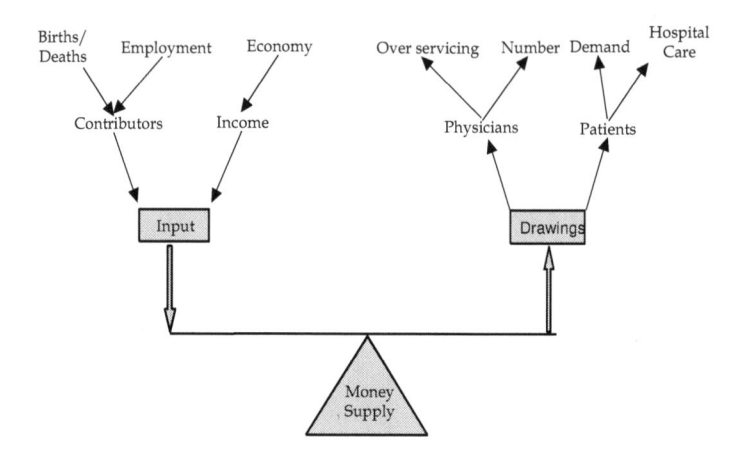

```
Births/
Deaths   Employment   Economy        Over servicing  Number  Demand  Hospital Care
    ↓        ↓           ↓                ↓            ↓       ↓        ↓
     Contributors      Income              Physicians          Patients
           ↓              ↓                     ↓                 ↓
              [Input]                              [Drawings]
                 ⇓                                     ⇑
                           △ Money Supply
```

The functional aspect in health care selected for scrutiny is the imbalance in cost. This is a design choice and does not address other imbalances such as inequity of delivery, although the two are probably closely intertwined. Stability ensues if the input of funding and drawings on the resulting money supply is equal, or if input exceeds drawings. If there is an increase in drawings, stability may be maintained by an increased input into the money supply. When this is no longer possible, and this is the case in health care, you have a mess. Rothman (1997) showed that the inflation rate in American health care (increased drawings) was above the national average for many decades. A growing economy helped to hide the potential instability until it came under strain itself, partly because of the health care cost problem. Hence, there is now both a decreased input and an increase in drawings (see **diagram 16**).

Input

Irrespective of the funding system (private, national health, or hybrid), those who contribute to the money supply are the employed. In other words, they subsidize the unemployed such as the young, the aged, and the disabled whether it is through taxation or medical insurance. An increase in the number of aged and a decrease in the number of births result in fewer contributors to the money supply. This is the situation in many First World countries. But an imbalance is also caused by an increase in the number of unemployed, or a reduced average income. Both these result from general economic or social factors. Economic imbalances are a fundamental problem in health care redesign in Third World countries where many of the population is unemployed or earn meager incomes. The burden on the employed becomes unbearable, particularly if the economy does not grow quickly enough in a sustainable manner.

Governments and businesses have a responsibility to institute and manage measures that will ensure employment and sustainable economic growth. Not only does this increase the money supply of the health care system, it also improves social conditions (housing, sewerage, feeding and literacy) and hence indirectly health. The first important intervention to restore balance in health care financing (and communal health) is therefore by government and business management of economic resources.

Drawings

The main reasons for the cost hemorrhage in health care were identified before. They may be grouped under two main headings, physicians (over supply and over servicing) and patients (increased demand and high technology hospital based care). The pressure on drawings is therefore created by the interaction between patient and physician. The patient-physician system is a highly complex decision-making interaction during which patient wants or needs is balanced with physician wants and ability, and is beyond the précis of the current discussion. It is the aim of most non-wholismic interventions to restore stability in health care funding by regulating this interaction. But the approaches are designed to control the structural problems identified only and ignore the mess as a whole. The result is likely to be an aggravation of the problem and not relief.

Controlling the cost spiral

Management science

To understand the management science approach towards the cost problem in health care, one has to understand that their philosophical foundation is a mixture of mechanismic and organismic thinking. They assume that illnesses are more or less the same in all patients and hence that treatment outcomes are predictable. Furthermore, they assume that all physicians, within narrow limits, have the same knowledge and abilities. The result of such thinking is a search for formulas for diagnosing and treating each illness with mathematical precision. If physicians can be convinced to practice according to a manual, like a manufacturing line in a plant, inputs and outputs and therefore cost can be controlled (managed). Hence it assumes that human activity and biological processes are machinelike (regular) and therefore controllable by persons qualified to manage (organismic thinking).

The management science position on cost is an assumption that cost is an environmental input and that control lies outside the system (mechanismic thinking). In other words, the health care delivery system has no reason to be directly involved in cost containment and the distribution of funds. Ideally, patients and physicians should be controlled from outside by government or administrators (Frankel, 1991; Hillman et al. 1992) according to a set of specifications to which the system should subscribe.

Quality Management

Quality Management for a while was considered to be a panacea for many of the problems of business management. Some authors suggested that it could also be applied to medical process to contain cost (Berwick, 1991; Laffel and Blumenthal, 1989). The idea is that through better knowledge of the customer, molding of the ideas of the organization, and increased control of the processes involved, the quality of care can be improved. The customer is considered to be an input and medical process the processing of the customer through the system.

Managed care

The business community uses Managed Care to pool consumer purchasing groups in order to contract for prepaid health care packages. The emphasis of this approach is on cost and there are fears that the probable effect could be a loss of quality (Holtgrewe, 1993; Levey and Hesse, 1985). The key constraint on physicians is a limitation on their autonomy of decision-making (Gruca and Nath, 1994; Iglehart, 1992b; Kongstvedt, 1989; Milstein et al. 1989) and for patients a closed panel of physicians to select from. Cost savings are achieved through control of physician income (salary or capitation) and a shift from hospital to ambulatory care (Gruca and Nath, 1994; Luft, 1978; Milstein et al. 1989). Physician decision-making is controlled by treatment and pre-admission protocols and a restricted medicines formulary, guided by various forms of medical audit (Milstein et al. 1989). In order to monitor utilization, a mushrooming bureaucracy is needed that forms a balancing loop with efforts to reduce cost (Grumet, 1989; Woolhandler and Himmelstein, 1991). In the USA, expenditure for health care administration accounts for 19 - 24% of the total health care budget (Saward, 1973) and the percentage is rising rapidly. The question is whether the army of bureaucrats offsets the modest saving from the elimination of unnecessary treatments (Woolhandler and Himmelstein, 1991). Managed Care is the fastest growing health care sector in the USA (Rothman, 1997).

The Department of Health, Education and Welfare originally prepared the Health Maintenance Organization (HMO) strategy for President Nixon during 1970. In his message to Congress, Nixon said that the purpose of

HMO's is to provide a strong financial incentive for better preventative care and greater efficiency (Saward, 1973). Some HMO's proved themselves to be efficient, but many less so, and none have been successful in the area of preventative care.

Managed Care *can* have an effect on cost control. The question is whether early gains will be sustained in the long-term (Teisberg and Porter, 1994). The experience with highly administered systems elsewhere seems to argue against this. There is now a patient and physician driven backlash in the USA against the managed care industry in the form of legislation, lawsuits, electoral-initiative drives, and negative media reporting (Bodenheimer, 1996). The issues underlying the backlash revolve, as can be predicted, around the following:

a) Restrictions on physician decision-making. Physicians are forbidden to recommend treatments that HMO's do not cover, and in some instances are paid bonuses for not recommending them. Physicians fiercely resist the system because of their loss of autonomy and status. Managers overcome the problem by importing more compliant physicians (enabled by the over supply of physicians), that in turn results in further resentment.
b) HMO's hire and retrench physicians for economic reasons, rather than clinical ineptness. The fear of retrenchment has a marked influence on physician behavior.
c) Selective contracting of physicians, in other words, the closed panel system. Many are willing to contract but are excluded from the system.
d) Gatekeeping. Delayed referral is leading to malpractice suits where HMO's are cited as the primary defendants.
e) The profit incentive. On the one hand, Managed Care denies patients treatments, but on the other pay physicians bonuses from profits accrued from the treatment withheld (according to Bodenheimer (1996), bonuses may add as much as 30 – 60% to a physician's salary). CEO's in Managed Care in the USA earn on average 62% more than their peers in other corporations of the same size. And finally, the Managed Care bureaucracy consumes 30% of patient contributions.
f) Managed Care plans are focused on healthy people with few health needs and avoid the chronically ill. The latter are left to fend for themselves or must join government plans in order to be cared for. The burden for dealing with those who contribute significantly to health care costs are therefore shifted to the state, who recover losses through taxation. Citizens in the end are no better off, only managed care is.

Audit
The study of the mistakes of treatment is part of the practice of medical audit, and one of the pillars of managed care. The focus is on physicians and the outcome of treatments (Brook and Lohr, 1985; Laffel and Blumenthal, 1989). The main objective of medical audit is to measure the quality of care (Lawrence, 1993). The underlying assumption is that it is possible to accurately measure the efficacy of treatment, which in turn assumes a linear cause-effect model (Brook and Lohr, 1985). It is also assumed that by collecting enough data, the final outcome of medical audit will be a comprehensive list of practice policies. The idea is that physicians will only have to look up a particular problem in a manual and then apply the formula with a guarantee that the problem will be successfully resolved (Eddy, 1990b). The assumption is that increasing precision can control cost, hence medical audit is founded on machine thinking.

A wholismic worldview on the other hand assumes high complexity with multiple co-producers and recursive causality. In a system where physicians have little control over process, the outcome of audit has to be considered very carefully in terms of the complexity of process and what may be happening, rather than what is assumed to be happening (Laffel and Blumenthal, 1989). Audit depends critically on selection criteria. This creates the usual dilemma, namely why these and not other criteria, who decides upon the criteria, and so on. In other words, it is a matter of the selection of co-producers and by definition important ones may be left out. Finally, according to Lomas et al. (1991), audit may have very little impact on the way that physicians behave and practice.

Risk management
The primary concern of risk management is the reduction of the effects of litigation on health care concerns (Mills and Von Bolschwing, 1995). It is defined as "a mechanism for managing exposure to risk that enables us to recognize the events that may result in unfortunate or damaging consequences in the future, their severity, and how they can be controlled". Or, more to the point, "the identification, analysis, and economic control of those risks which can threaten the *assets* or *earning capacity* of an enterprise" (Dickson, 1995). It implies:

a) The identification of risk.
b) That the eventual control mechanism must be *economic*.
c) The protection of the *means* of an organization.
d) It has its origins in manufacturing or process industries, the principles of which are directly extrapolated to service industries.
e) Measures that will protect the objectives of an enterprise in other words *profit*.

Risk management consists of two activities, risk analysis, during which the economic impacts of risk is analyzed, and risk control, that is the process of economic control. The latter entails steps to prevent adverse events and the reduction of the impact once it occurs. Using this information, a decision is made whether the organization should transfer the risk, that is insure itself against it, or retain the risk, in other words accept that it is less expensive to settle adverse events out of profits. The approach is value-free.

In practice, risk management attempts to alter physician behavior by using the traditional methods of learning associated with management science (Moss, 1995). The focus is on maximizing quality of care by using clinical audit. The idea is that the activity of audit will lead to self-reflection and therefore learning. The problem is how does one determine what is quality medical care? More importantly, a study of human errors in complex environments shows that most errors are in fact messes caused by the confluence of a number of decisions, often separated from each other in time. In problem systems, the individual at the "coal face" is often blamed for the error, but in reality bears the brunt for existing weakness in the system. Sadly, legal blame apportion is based upon a similar simple linear model of causality where medical errors are concerned.

Adverse events (AE), in other words unintended injury caused by treatment that lead to increased hospital stay or disability at the time of discharge occurs in about 4% of hospital admissions (Leape, 1994). This translates into approximately 98 000 adverse events (AE) per year in New York state alone. Of these, 14% of patients die as a result of their injuries and 7% have a prolonged or permanent disability. About 70% of AE's are found to be preventable and of them, 44% are the result of technical errors, 17% diagnostic errors, and 10% drug related. Only 20% of technical errors are deemed to be the result of negligence, but in the case of diagnostic errors, the figure rises to 71%. Technical errors are likely to be the result of a lack of skills or experience (poor or incorrect education), diagnostic errors the result of lack of knowledge, experience, or incorrect analysis (decision-making), and errors in drug use a lack of communication in the hospital system.

In reality, human errors are a rare event as compared with successes or correct actions. Most tasks require the use of knowledge for problem solving, and the translation of knowledge into action (implementation) is one of the most vulnerable actions to error in human activity systems (Van Cott, 1994). People tend to avoid reasoning their way to solutions and instead tend to use one of two mechanisms for complex problem solving, similarity matching, or frequency gambling (Moray, 1994). This means that people will decide that a present situation resembles one that occurred before, or, faced with uncertainty, a course of action will be selected that worked before.

A major risk factor in the cause of medical errors is the complexity of modern health care systems (Leape, 1994). For example, in an average sized 600-bed teaching hospital in the USA, approximately 4 million doses of drugs are administered per year. If the system was 99,9% error free, which it is not, it would still translate into 4 000 errors per year. If it is accepted that errors are unavoidable in complex human activity systems such as the health care system, efforts to reduce iatrogenic injuries must focus on the systemic nature of such errors.

Government

The state traditionally addresses problems by setting up commissions of inquiry. Take for example the Agency for Health Care Policy and Research (in 1989) in the USA. The object of this agency was to investigate how the databases of hospitals and health insurance organizations could be used to determine the efficiency of treatments (an objective similar to clinical audit). It is now accepted that the Patient Outcomes Research Teams (PORTS) set up to investigate the agreed upon topics yielded no data of any significance (Kingman, 1994). The reasons from a systems perspective are not difficult to determine. It is assumed that the databases are correct and complete. Nothing could be further from the truth. The information on claims forms (diagnoses, treatment given, and so on) only reflects what physicians want it to reflect. The fact is that one has to enter a diagnosis or code on a form in order to be reimbursed. These forms do not allow for multiple or complex diagnoses. Furthermore, the code determines the tariff of payment and there is a well known but unstated incentive to "pad" such codes (Milstein et al. 1989).

Secondly, governments attempt to regulate or control health care systems as a whole. A recent example is the ANC Health Plan for South Africa (Anonymous, 1994b). To government, the ideal form of control is to install its own bureaucracy to manage the system and in particular to collect and distribute funding through an NHS plan (Benatar, 1985; De Beer and Broomberg, 1990). This approach does not take into account the possible effects of such intervention on the system as a whole and also other systems with which it interacts. Not only is the health care system changed irretrievably, but also other industries such as the pharmaceutical industry may disappear, which will influence employment, government revenue, and eventually health care funding. This could lead to a reinforcing loop that will doom the health care system to mediocrity.

The NHS system is an attempt to control patient and physician behavior by regulating the health care environment. Employment contracts spell out salaried physicians' relationship with the employer (government). Treatment choice is restricted by a medicines formulary (which indirectly controls the pharmaceutical industry), and by regulating hospitals, in other words, the treatment environment. Patients, as in managed care, are denied a free choice of physician. Government control does not appear to influence the patient-physician interaction, which may be one reason why the electorate is often not dissatisfied with the model.

Physicians in NHS systems are traditionally poorly remunerated. The result is a lack of incentive and long waiting lists. In 1979, 31% of the 556 000 patients awaiting surgery of all kinds in Britain had been waiting for more than a year (Schwartz and Aaron, 1984). Of urgent cases (which represent 7% of waiting cases), 75% had been waiting for more than a month. Waiting lists leads to pressure for a private health care system.

NHS models are funded by income tax contributions, which has two effects. Firstly, the cost of health care becomes "hidden" in the budget as a whole and increasing demand for health care is funded by raising taxes. Voters are usually uninformed about the specific effect of the health care budget on the increase consequently they have no understanding of how their behavior affects the health care system and ultimately their tax contribution. Secondly, health care has to compete with other social priorities for expenditures under public review (Saward, 1973). There can never be enough funds for health care on its own and the situation is likely to deteriorate in time. In the long term, this problem can only be resolved by an approach that is able to engender understanding of the social system as a whole, and more importantly, of the importance of social responsibility.

Historically, on many occasions government intervention had unforeseen effects on the system as a whole. For example, changes in the NHS in Britain led to a reduced number of referrals to teaching hospitals, with subsequent damage to research and teaching (Mundell, 1992). In Zimbabwe, a primary care rural network was started but due to economic factors in other systems that were ignored, the system is on the verge of collapse (Logie, 1993). The Swedish NHS failed and primary health care is now being remodeled into a partially free market, free choice system again (Nilsson, 1993). In Germany, a new law was introduced to curb the prescription of drugs. Physicians are expected to cover any excess if the drug budget is exceeded. As a result of this law, physicians are afraid of losing income and consequently under prescribe. Not only are patients unhappy about this but also pharmaceutical companies are suffering severe losses (Tuffs, 1993) and government is losing revenue. The consequence is pressure on the government by the pharmaceutical industry to rescind their decision in order to save their investments.

Regulation affects the ability of organizations to adapt to a changing environment (Gruca and Nath, 1994). The regulations themselves often create external constraints that may either limit the ability to adapt, or lead to misalignment with the environment that makes survival impossible. For example, constraints introduced by government to regulate the treatment of Medicare patients in hospitals in the USA makes it impossible for these institutions to recover the losses that they suffer. The burden for the loss in revenue is therefore shifted to private paying patients. The result is a situation where private patients can no longer afford hospital care and hospitals with an insufficient number of privately funded patients can no longer survive and have to close down. In the end, Medicare patients are left without a hospital to attend at all. The government decision created a reinforcing causality loop that damaged the system as a whole.

Illich (1976) quotes another classic example of how government intervention created a problem. In Borneo, villagers were bitten by malaria carrying mosquitoes. The resulting malaria epidemic caused villagers to approach their elected representatives (politicians), who called in the "experts". They determined that DDT would be the most efficient way to exterminate the mosquitoes. The air force was ordered to spray the forests. Shortly afterwards, a bubonic plague epidemic broke out in the villages. It subsequently turned out that DDT contaminates cockroaches (who are mostly resistant to its effects) that is part of the diet of geckoes. Geckoes became lethargic from the DDT and hence easy prey for cats. The latter are highly susceptible to and died from DDT poisoning, resulting in an increased number of rats hence bubonic plague. The army had to parachute cats into the jungle to save the villagers. The experts neglected the whole and the environment that would be affected by the DDT and their actions. Modern governments, in dealing with health care, show no signs of learning from past mistakes.

An important problem with attempts of governments to control the behavior of individuals is increased numbers of rules (laws), which clutter the decision-making environment. The result is increased complexity (Moray, 1994), increased risk for more errors, which requires more rules, and so on.

Government is an important co-producer to the health care system and often represents the wishes of the electorate. As such, it is in a position of power not only to affect the system, but also to change it. The question is, can they contribute to better health care systems in a way that may improve the health care and health care delivery of all its citizens, or are they irretrievably locked into the expediency of doing whatever it takes to get re-elected?

The medical profession

Recommendations from the profession itself have been few and in general, as to be expected, are aimed at maintaining the status quo, in other words to protect profits (Scott and Shapiro, 1992). Sadly, the medical profession has forgotten its obligation to society, i.e. the system of which it is a part and that is responsible for its continued existence.

The social sciences

Social science contributes mostly towards the philosophy of health planning. Two streams of thought will be discussed briefly as an example.

Some authors suggest that the right to health care ought to be a fundamental point of departure for planning (Van Rensburg and Fourie, 1993; Van Rensburg and Fourie, 1994). This is an idealistic position with a problematic transition to pragmatic implementable plans. Social science often concerns itself with the design of philosophical ideologies for political intervention, but not with the practical implications of intervention. Politicians as the most likely decision-makers and implementers are often attracted to such ideas.

Ivan Illich (1976) argues that society transferred the power to determine illness and the rules according to which it will be dealt with to the medical profession. The result is exploitation of patients and a position of privilege for physicians. Curative medicine contributed very little towards improving the health of mankind, on the contrary, many illnesses is caused by medical intervention. In general, the largest contribution towards health is through better housing and nutrition. To Illich, the solution lies therein that the laity should want to care for themselves again and that constitutional limits should be placed on the health care system, in other words political control.

An important social role of physicians is to assign people to different social categories. For example, they decide who may stay away from work, who may be soldiers, who are insane, and so on. As a result, between 15 - 30% of consultations are for obtaining sick notes. In addition, physicians are trained to do something and therefore are biased to diagnose, even though that may be unnecessary. This system implies a standard of normality against which people may be measured, any deviance from which is considered pathological and hence something must be done about it.

The health care system caused a change in society's worldviews of pain, sickness, suffering and dying. Today, in most first world countries, these issues are considered to be unnatural, in other words, the health care system removed from their communities the meaning and ability to deal with and tolerate them. Whereas pain and suffering and the ability to deal with it in a dignified manner was considered to be an inevitable component of life in the past, today these sensations when present are considered to be a failure of the health care system. This implies that the meaning of and response to illness is a socially created reality, and hence, since the health care system is a reflection of the social and cultural values of society (Saward, 1973), is an expression of our cultural history. An extension of this argument is that the image of death of a society determines a culture's image of health. Whereas in the past, death was considered to be a natural phenomenon, the modern concept is dominated by the idea of natural death. This means that dying from an unnatural cause (such as illness), before a yardstick determined by medical science is reached is unnatural. Physicians and patients therefore came to believe that the former have power over death and dying and if someone dies before the allotted time, someone has erred and must be punished.

> "*Socially approved death happens when man has become useless not only as a producer but also as a consumer. It is the point at which a consumer, trained at great expense, must finally be written off as a total loss. Dying has become the ultimate form of consumer resistance*" (Illich, 1976).

The trouble with Illich's approach is that a return to a natural state (the past) is utopian and probably impossible. It seems senseless to deny available sources of knowledge about health. More importantly, how can they be used more efficiently? His crucial insight is the need for greater patient participation in health care matters and the identification of "health" as a construct of social interaction. As an indictment against modern medicine, Illich's work is of monumental importance and ought to be a source of reflection to the health care system.

The systems community

Attempts to remodel health care by the systems community shows remarkable naivety and is dogged by a lack of understanding and attention to the complexity of medical process. Berwick (1994) correctly identifies the need for greater learning about health care matters at the level of local communities. He identifies the criteria for a health care learning system as, efficient leadership to ensure implementation, employee participation, encouragement of employees to be creative, and attempts to understand community needs. The approach in the main is organismic, hence the need for leadership (a brain for thinking) and employee participation (for feedback). Its only concession to wholism is acceptance that hospital based health care is embedded in a social environment, that is, the larger whole. The learning system approach as used by Berwick does nothing towards stabilizing the mess in health care. Gregory et al. (1995) participated in a study to determine the need for greater user participation in defining quality standards within the NHS. Again the underlying assumption is organismic, that is, it is possible to determine standards of health care behavior and the fundamental concept of "health" remains unchallenged. Hence, by implication, it accepts uncritically the entrenched health care system, as it exists. Gregory's then is an attempt to wrap medical audit in a systems blanket. Rovin et al. (1994) applied interactive planning to design an idealized health care system for the U.S.A. Surprisingly, again the concept of "health" as ultimate purpose of the system goes unchallenged. Consequently, there is no attention to the redesign of medical process to achieve the ideal. An interesting suggestion is a government mandated coupon type of payment system. Dodds (1993) also used interactive planning as basis for a participative approach to a local community clinic. The intervention accepted the constraints of the traditional socio-medical political structures within which the community and clinic is embedded, hence change is possible only on a local and very limited scale.

Ulrich's (1994b) is a critique of health care planning, using the planning of the Areawide Health System Agency of Puget Sound to show up the deceptions that occur when the health care environment is ignored. In other words, health planning cannot be about health services only. Since planning (and in this instance health planning) is a design for a purposeful social (human activity) system, planning for health should be to improve "health". The assumptions we make about "health" are a source of deception if not reflected upon, and consequently the concept ought to include the totality of the aspects that constitute "health". I submit that this insight is of critical importance for health care planning. Ulrich closely follows Illich's understanding of the concept of "health". Idealized health design then, ought to be based upon:

a) Minimizing dependency on professionally delivered health care by,
   i) Improving quality of life through the environment, and
   ii) Encouraging self-care.
b) Healthcare delivery compatible with the aims of self-care.

It is on this critical issue that Ulrich himself is deceived. Like Illich, he ignores the fact that health care delivery is the historical product of a communal need for health care professionals. The scientific-technological complex disturbed, or one may even say destroyed, the stability of this important social function. Furthermore, by minimizing (read avoid) or detaching contact with what in the end is a communally acquired knowledge base, stability is not restored it is disturbed even more. My understanding of social stability is as described by Vickers (1984). The route to reliable, accessible, equitable, participative and affordable health care is more likely to be by improving the interface between patient and physician than, in the manner of managed care gatekeeping, widening it.

According to Ulrich, health planning is a political act with redistributive effects and ethical implications, hence requires a collective basis of legitimization. He identifies the key client of planning as those most helpless to cope with suffering and illness, the poor, the old, the uneducated, the working class, the unemployed and the unemployable, in other words the socially disadvantaged. This appears to be based on an assumption that people are disadvantaged as a result of circumstance, that is because of an unfavorable environment created by others and that people have no personal choice. Not only would such an assumption be difficult to defend in terms of actual human behavior, but it also suggests a notion of control more compatible with mechanismic or organismic thinking than wholism. Additionally, Ulrich appears to suggest that those who are not the main client but likely to be affected by planning (or their witnesses), ought to participate in design. In this case it could be physicians and they could be asked to participate in actions that are likely to disadvantage themselves. Not only would that be coercive, but it also begs the question, what will guarantee their co-operation, given that they will have to live the consequences of redistribution? In other words, to raise another wholismic issue, what guarantees the implementation of planning? That irrespective of the owner of the system health care funding is redistributive is a reality that was referred to earlier and that appears to have been ignored by Ulrich as well. In summary then, Ulrich raises the quality of debate to a higher level, but in the end ignores important aspects of the whole.

Henrik Blum's (1983) work[1] is a valuable contribution towards health care planning in a wholismic fashion. His approach is to generate a systemic understanding of what produces good "health" and what is socially desirable, and from this he deducts what is required in terms of institutions, relationships, services, and individual participation. According to him, illness is the result of a disturbance in the relationship between individual and environment. "Health" then is the state in which the individual does the best with the capabilities available to him or her. The emphasis of health care delivery then is to assist people to adjust their behavior towards more "healthy" living. The basis on which health care delivery ought to be designed is participative decision-making, personal liberty, equal opportunity, and equal access. In practice, this results in a combination of traditional medical care, self-care and collective activities towards a healthier environment. His system requires a national health policy, redesign of traditional physician training and national financing funded from taxation. Churchman influenced Blum, as can be seen from his commitment to equity and participation. Blum's study then, is the only one that could substantially assist in the resolution of the mess, but in common with the others, does not question the fundamental assumptions made about "health" and purpose. Apart from Blum, a deprivation model of illness is still in vogue as the basis for planning as illustrated by the studies quoted, and the poverty of deprivation as model itself is a significant part of the problem.

---

[1] Blum, a health planner, worked closely with Churchman at the University of California Berkeley.

What lessons from the mess?

What can we learn from conceptualizing the cost crisis in health care as a mess? Any planned intervention that does not take cognizance of the problem situation as a whole is likely to postpone the inevitable at best, or to result in a further deterioration at worst. Systems or wholes are complex, unpredictable, and as a result, the concept of control has little meaning. Successful interventions will most likely have to address the following aspects identified as important, both from the system dynamics model of the mess and efforts to stabilize the cost problem in health care.

   a) Ownership of the system. Most systems methodologies identify participation in planning as vital to change and implementation (see for instance Rovin, Dodds, and Ulrich). Managed Care and government intervention, in the end hand fails because it is fundamentally coercive and characterized by a lack of participation. Until now, the wishes of both patients and physicians, in other words of those affected by planning, were universally ignored. Some concession is made to patient participation by social science planning (Illich) and attempts at wholismic intervention (Rovin, Dodds, and Ulrich), but physicians are left without a witness.
   b) Those interventions most likely to restore balance in the mess will alter patient and physician behavior in a non-coercive fashion. The ideal towards which behavior ought to be adjusted depends critically on the communal concept of "health" and to be useful, the model has to be wholismic. If it is a potentially affordable concept, then there are numerous ways in which behavior may be guided towards a socially acceptable health system.
   c) As recognized by Ulrich, the mind map of "health". "Health" is a symbolic system and product of social interaction (Ulrich, 1994b). Hence, it has a history, depends on the perceptions of local communities, and is in constant evolution. The prevailing concept of "health" does not accurately reflect physical reality (see White quoted in McWhinney (1981)), and hence is an important co-producer of the mess. The ways we conceptualize "health" determines patient wants and needs, and also patient and physician behavior. All planning until now assumed "health" to be a simple and easily determinable parameter, that there is consensus about its meaning, and therefore something that may be safely ignored. Not questioning the purpose and very foundation of health care is an important omission of all health planning (Ulrich, 1994b).
   d) Decision-making. Diagnosis and treatment decisions are both generated by and hence products of the patient-physician interaction. But more importantly, these decisions set in motion those processes that will eventually have to be remunerated, hence are the basic

activity affecting the cost spiral. Effective medical decision-making depends on the quality of available knowledge and the mind map of "health" within which it is framed. Both are amenable to change and cost-effective behavior from both patients and physicians is therefore the simplest and potentially most powerful measure to stabilize the mess. Because of the complexity of human systems, there is a wide range of error and difference in decision-making styles. In common with all complex systems, the variation is difficult to control. Managed care and government planners, as shown earlier, believe that the decision-making environment may be controlled, using measures that are often perceived as coercive. The cause of the error is machine and organismic thinking.

e) Physician reward system. At the moment, physicians are rewarded for behavior that will maximize profits (an economic model). The reward system ought to be changed to reward the efficient use of skills and knowledge, in other words, cost-effective behavior (a behavioral model). This becomes possible if the mind map of "health" is altered and medical process adjusted accordingly.

f) Efficient use of knowledge. In a profit maximizing system physicians have an incentive to hoard the product they sell, which is knowledge. In a system geared towards greater efficiency, knowledge is shared; hence better decision-making and less cost. The aim of design should not be to dissociate patients from knowledge by gatekeeping and self-care, but to use available knowledge more efficiently. According to Toffler (1990), we are in a transition from the technological to the information age, disowning the reality does not prevent it from happening.

The mechanismic and organismic worldviews conceptualize the organization of human activity simplistically. However, intervention based on simplistic notions in highly complex and finely balanced systems often have unforeseen and unwanted results. Neglecting to consider all aspects of the decision-making environment of health care, as Ulrich showed, is a source of deception and error. It is apparent from this study that efforts at health care redesign, both from wholismic and non-wholismic sources are based on incorrect assumptions about important aspects of the problem situation. The result is that in common with all complex systems, understanding of the whole, hence in this example the cost crisis in health care is lost. Health care is not only a mess, it is a system and the only possible avenue for restoring stability to the cost problem is by a systems approach. Using such an approach, meaningful participation in design by patients and physicians becomes possible with an improved possibility that planned changes to the system will be implemented. In addition, those who affect and are affected by the system may learn how their behavior affects the whole.

In summary, this chapter investigated the question *"why is there a problem situation?"* Investigation revealed that although current attempts at problem solving are based upon an assumption of simple linear processes, the health care system is a complex human activity system composed of multiple interactive processes linked by complex causal interactions. Attempts to alter the system have not met with much success, since they do not take the complexity of such systems into consideration. Intervention in complex systems often can and does result in unintended effects on other components of the system. I submit that a change in the image that health care planners have about health care, could have a positive effect on future health care planning.

In order to answer the question *"how did the problem arise?"* the historic development of the health care system has to be studied. This will be the focus of the argument in the next chapter.

Chapter 7: An Archaeology Of The Problem Situation

The health care system exists because society has a need for people with special knowledge to deal with illness when society is no longer able to do so itself (Saward, 1973). The structure of the health care system today is linked inseparably to its historic development, and to understand the structure and process of health care, we therefore have to examine its history.

Historically, the health care system grew from a simple interaction between patients and physicians into a complex social system with multiple interactions. This was caused mostly as a result of human intervention and the outcome was unforeseen interactions, often with unsatisfactory consequences for the system as a whole. The problem is that man's ability to intervene did not equal the ability to control the outcomes. The reason for this development is that increased knowledge resulted in a need for more complex models of illness, and therefore treatment of a higher order of complexity. Such treatments necessitated in the introduction of more professionals (specialists), both physicians and other health care workers, into the system and therefore an increase in the number of social interactions necessary to give medical treatments. The problem is that that both illness and medical process are still perceived as simple uncomplicated processes.

In ancient times health was associated almost exclusively with our mentally created universe. Modern medicine attempts to shift the emphasis to science and therefore the physical universe. However, the mind map we have of illness, health, the role of physicians and even many of the problems that we experience as ill health still belongs to the former. The trouble is that it is in this arena that wants are created, wants that in many cases we can no longer afford. Changing mind maps may lead to aligned self-control and therefore a more efficient and affordable health care system.

History Of The Patient-Physician Interaction[1]

For the purpose of this book, the history of medicine will be classified as follows:

---

[1]Chamberlain and Ogilvie, 1974, Haeger, 1988; Singer, 1961

1. The pre-scientific (ancient) era.
2. The scientific era
    2.1 Pre-renaissance.
    2.2 Post-renaissance.
3. Technological era.
4. Information era.

This classification follows an increase in complexity of the interaction between the different components of the system. It also follows the history of Western philosophy.

Pre-scientific (ancient) era

This era is arbitrarily taken to be the time before the rise of Greek philosophy with its subsequent influence on the development of Western culture. It is also the time that 'primitive' medicine was practiced, with an emphasis on intuition and ritual rather than empirical method. In fact, until the 18th Century, physicians only talked to patients, they did not examine them (Kriel, 1996). The practice of medicine associated with this era is essentially still being practiced today in parts of Africa, Asia and South America. The implication is that although those systems did not escape the influence of Western culture and Western medicine, it is still bound by the conventions that it originated from. It will be shown that these assumptions inevitably lead to a difference in both the perception and experience of the medical process by different cultures[2]. It follows that it also has an important bearing on the patient-physician interaction.

The physician

Members of society will usually attempt to deal with illness themselves until a point is reached where they lack the knowledge and skills to do so. The need arose in primitive societies for individuals prepared to overcome this barrier by collecting available knowledge about illness and who could be consulted in time of need. Historically, some members of the community felt themselves called to heal and would apply to and be accepted by existing practitioners of the art for training[3]. Training would be by way of an apprenticeship, which sometimes took many years and would mostly be practical. (Medical training is in effect still an apprenticeship, but the basic training follows the conventions of modern university training). Students

---

[2] See Foucault, quoted in Illich (1976).
[3] We still have to apply for and must be selected for medical training. In the ancient era, physicians decided who would be suitable candidates for training. Today, educators make that decision. This has an important bearing on the kind of person allowed to become part of the community of physicians and may be part of the problem in modern health care.

would be instructed not only in recognizing different illnesses and their causes, but also in finding the ingredients for making up medications and how they should be prescribed. The secrets of the profession were handed down from teacher to pupil by way of an oral tradition, the origins of treatments coming from the forgotten past. The practice of an apprenticeship was continued in Western medicine by the guild of barber-surgeons (McWhinney, 1989)[4].

After the successful completion of training, in some societies the new professionals would be publicly initiated so that everyone could recognize their standing in society as professionals. This ritual is still practiced in modern medicine in the form of the Oath that all medical students swear to in public at the time of their graduation. This is society's way of confirming the healer's position as a professional and expert. In modern society, this position is also codified by the physician's acceptance by and registration with a medical council. Such councils are statutory bodies and serve as a barrier of entrance into the profession. They are appointed and supported by the state and control therefore rests with government.

The practice[5]

Traditional healers often formed societies or associations amongst themselves in their communities. It was accepted that these professionals would be reimbursed for practicing their trade, but they were also trusted not to be exorbitant in their request for remuneration. Those with special skills had a high standing in society and were able to earn well (Haeger, 1988).

According to Mbiti (1971)

> "These people have a language, symbolism, knowledge, skill, practice and what I may call 'office personality' of their own, which are not known or easily accessible to the ordinary person"

This perception of the profession still underlies assumptions about the interactions in modern health care systems. Patients have an image of a physician's "bedside manner", a metaphysical idea that is impossible to define. It is a sought after attribute and contributes to the professional image and standing of the physician.

---

[4]The modern relics of the barber's pole (the red line of blood from blood letting) and the habit of calling specialist surgeons mister originate from them. Physicians trained at universities and could therefore lay claim to the title doctor. Surgeons were apprenticed and belonged to a guild of barber-surgeons and consequently could not.
[5]The following discussion is based upon healing as practised as part of African culture.

The fundamental distinguishing feature of this era is a "holistic" approach. It was thought that illness sis caused by the ill will of other people, or by the spirits through witchcraft or sorcery. To treat such illnesses required that the traditional healer not only diagnose and treat, but also deal with the spiritual aspect of the illness. Therefore in African villages, even today disease and misfortune are religious experiences and require a religious approach to deal with them.

> "*They (healers) have access to the force of nature and other forms of knowledge unknown or little known by the public*" (Mbiti, 1971).

The public entrusted them with the duty of removing that, which may be harmful to the community. The idea about the mystical power of healers is the source of an extraordinary trust in medical practitioners, even today. It also says something about the close relationship between healers and the communities that they were part of, relationships that are disturbed in modern society.

Traditional healers symbolized the *hopes* of society: hopes of good health, protection and security from evil forces, prosperity and good fortune and ritual cleansing when harm or impurities were contracted. This understanding became part of the collective subconscious in the West and has important implications for the way that modern patients perceive their diagnosis and treatment. The question is, does the modern physician still satisfy the community's need for protection from misfortune?

Traditional healers are clothed in the regalia of their profession, such as animal skins and so on. In modern medicine, physicians are identified by the white coats they wear.

Ethics

The concept that physicians should act ethically in relation to their community is a very old one. The first known code of conduct dates back to 2000 BC in Babylon (Code of Hammurabi). This Code determined that physicians could determine remuneration according to a patient's social status, but also that they would be legally accountable for poor treatment (De Wet, 1991; Haeger, 1988). The problem of a fair profit and accountability therefore is a very old one, and the Oath ascribed to in modern medicine is still an expression of the moral principles that reflect the major beliefs of the society that physicians serve (Pellegrino, 1976).

The concept of professionals as people in possession of special knowledge and skills also stems from this time and is fundamental to many modern day assumptions, as will be shown later.

The ancient beliefs, although very much submerged in the collective subconscious of society (in a Jungian sense) is still very much central to the wants and expectations of patients in their interaction with the medical profession. This is not surprising, considering the fact that they are an integral historic part of belief systems about illness and health, and were altered by the appreciative systems of society into the modern version. After the ancient era, the development of the medical profession became a product of our Western culture, African and Eastern cultures having retained the essence of the ancient era. The fundamental approach of this time is more systemic than today but also spiritually weighted or intuitive. The concept of illness and the recommended treatment is based upon a perception of the mind and the working of primitive reason and therefore a primitive image of illness.

Scientific era

Pre-renaissance

During this period the ideas of the Greek philosophers started to influence the practice of medicine and by tradition the school of Hippocrates of Cos (460 - 377 BC) is usually credited for this. Hippocrates' contribution is not that of improved treatment or even the understanding of illness to the profession, but he introduced the concept of *observation* into the medical armamentarium[6]. This means the empirical observation of illness (De Wet, 1991), its symptoms and signs, and its course, rather than a reliance on the assumption of vapors and humors as the cause of illness. The direct result of this is that this period signaled the start of increased empirical learning about illness and its causes. These schools continued throughout the Middle Ages (frequently under the auspices of the Church) and changed little until the start of the reformation. As a result of this approach medicine became less religious and more scientific. The cause of illness was no longer in the environment of the patient but came from the body. The physician subsequently became more aware of the body as a vessel containing illness. Presumably it also meant that although reason in the form of the rationalistic tradition was still an integral part of the concept of illness, empirical ideas started to permeate the practice of physicians through the process of observation and reflection of what the senses perceived. Today there has almost been an over correction in the sense that the body being treated is no longer part of the patient.

An important contribution to the art of medicine was made during this period by the contact with the Moorish (Arabian) culture, whose medical

---

[6]The resources available to a person engaged in a task (Allen, 1992).

expertise and knowledge at that point in time was further advanced than that of their Western counterparts.

Hippocrates also contributed to modern medicine his famous Oath. This document emphasizes the individuality of the patient, a commitment from physicians to help their patients and *to do no harm* to them. The latter is an important position virtually forgotten today.

Post-renaissance

During the renaissance the idea of empirical observation was further developed. In medicine, the work of Andreas Vesalius (ca 1543) acted as a stimulus for the rekindling of growth in the profession. He rewrote the dormant discipline of anatomy based upon his observations of the anatomy of animals. This questioned many of the commonly held assumptions about disease processes believed in until then. The newfound knowledge permeated the world, thanks to the discovery of the printing press. It now became possible for anyone who could read to study the published texts. One therefore no longer had to be apprenticed to gain access to knowledge and in this case medical knowledge. From now on, as in the case of religion with the translation and printing of the bible, lay people would be able to read and gain some knowledge about their illness. The expertise of physicians was no longer theirs and theirs alone. Patients started to interact with physicians if they had the opportunity to learn about their bodies and wanted to do so. Illness was no longer a religious experience or an interest of the community in the religious sense. However, all information disseminated in this way was not accurate, a problem that is still apparent in the lay press today. The problem with this is that misrepresentations, even unintentional ones, have the ability to shape the image of patients of illness, health and the health care system, and these images can sometimes have serious results.

Until now the physical examination depended on the unaided senses. The introduction of the stethoscope, thermometer, and so on as aids to diagnosis helped the expansion of knowledge about disease and also the process of diagnosis and treatment during the eighteenth century (Chamberlain and Ogilvie, 1974). In addition, developments in the fields of chemistry, physics and astronomy, lead to the development of disciplines such as bacteriology, radiology, endocrinology, and so on. They not only added to the knowledge of disease, but also to the process of diagnosis and treatment (McWhinney, 1989). From now on the traditional process of diagnosis and treatment was formulated in the form in which it essentially is still used today, namely:

- History taking.
- Physical examination.
    a) Observation.
    b) Palpation.

- c) Percussion.
- d) Auscultation.
* Differential diagnosis.
* Special examinations.
* Diagnosis.
* Treatment.

This was the era where the concept of the *clinician* was born (literally bedside art (Allen, 1992)). They were people known for their ability to make an excellent diagnosis by the use of observation and deduction. Modern patients still have this image as part of their imagery of how a physician should be and act. The image of the professional was altered and expanded during this time. This is partly explained by the fact that in the 17th and 18th Centuries physicians were a small group of learned individuals educated in a few universities (McWhinney, 1989). They practiced mainly in towns amongst the rich and influential, a practice that is still followed today. One of the fundamental problems of the health care system still is a preponderance of practitioners in cities and wealthier areas with a relative shortage amongst poor and rural communities.

The empirical knowledge of medicine now grew exponentially. It was the time when observation of patients and their problems and the interpretation thereof came to the fore. Their rapidly changing environment largely drove the growth and change in the medical profession. One can ask the question whether the knowledge of medicine as a discipline grew by itself or whether knowledge grew as a result of growth in the related disciplines such as chemistry, biochemistry, anatomy, and so on, and medicine just borrowed from it. From a systems point of view, it may be more correct to say that medicine is a product of the interaction with its environment, i.e. both the health care system and the environment influenced and changed each other. This point may be more than merely of academic interest.

According to Kuhn (1962), the principal reason for the existence of the professions is social need. His method, the examination of science by its historical data, recognizes the development of mature science by the successive transition from one paradigm via revolution to another. He postulates that a science is pre-scientific if it merely gathers facts and in the absence of an implicit body of beliefs in the discipline has to have one supplied by another discipline. By this definition medicine is a pre-scientific discipline and not a science in the sense that Kuhn defined it. In terms of this definition, medicine is not a discipline with a clear paradigm. A review of the published literature is more that of the reporting of factual data than speculation, which by Kuhn's definition proves this point. It would be fair to say that modern medicine took on the worldview of Newtonian science with its separation of the observer from the observed (Kriel, 1996), in other words, a mechanismic model of illness and health care. This has important implications for the way that the practitioners of the craft form their belief systems about the body of work that they use to practice with.

The increase in knowledge in health care systems resulted in an increased need by the system for specialists, which resulted in more components added to the system and more complex and intricate interactions. Physicians became busier with their newfound diagnostic tools and the discoveries in botany, chemistry, etc., contributed to the complexity of the pharmaceutical field. The potions to be used were handed over to the chemist to prepare and distribute. At first, the ill were treated at home where they were visited and treated by physicians and their assistants making "house calls". (The concept of home care is still an important issue in health care today). Later, those in need were cared for in temples, monasteries and sick houses[7] by what later became the professional nurse. By the 18th Century, the emphasis of hospital care changed from care for the incurable, sick poor and disabled, to the curable sick. This trend was accelerated by specialization and the need to use special apparatus for diagnosis and treatment, which could only be found in hospitals (Knowles, 1973). Patients were now removed from their homes to a hospital, where they were nursed under the supervision of the physician. The nursing profession became of age through the efforts of Florence Nightingale during the Crimean War. These additions to health care, the chemist, the nurse and the hospital, were the start of a rapidly increasing number of interactions and subsequent complexity in the health care environment in which the patient-physician interaction takes place. The original interaction involved two people, the physician and the patient, and an embracing environment. Now the interaction involved four groups of people, the physician, the patient, the hospital system (including nursing care), and the pharmacist. The observation to be made though is that physicians were still considered by tradition to be the directors of the orchestra (the brain) and therefore had to be "in charge" and make the decisions. The concept of being in charge is still an important part of the modern image that both patients and physicians have of medical practitioners. In addition, as a result of this, it is believed that they are responsible for all the actions and interactions that take place in the "orchestra" and that they are in control.

Technological era

This period can roughly be taken to follow the industrial revolution. People now started to substitute machines to do work for them (Ackoff, 1981). In medicine this period saw the introduction of highly sophisticated equipment to aid in diagnosis and treatment. It was the time of advances such as X-rays, anesthetics, the discovery of insulin and penicillin, and so on. The

---

[7]The word hospital comes from the Latin *hospes*, which means guest, or host. The words hostel and hotel are derived from the same root (Knowles, 1973).

introduction of technology had a profound and systemic impact, and contributes to the current crisis in the profession. This period resulted in an explosion of knowledge. Not only did more knowledge become available to the physician, but also many previously unheard of, sophisticated treatments became possible. This by necessity impacted on the wants of patients[8]. In many instances discoveries were driven by the wants of society and not their needs. This resulted in strains not only on delivery systems and costs, but (some may say more importantly) traditional values and ethical systems of society and medicine were put under increasing strain (De Wet, 1991; Claassen and Verschoor, 1992).

The knowledge load became such that individual physicians could not hope to know everything about their discipline any longer (Grant and Dixon, 1987), which lead to the introduction of the specialist into the system. Pediatrics was the first separately recognized discipline in the USA (in 1892) and the major disciplines all came into existence during the first part of the 20th Century. Further fragmentation into sub-specialties started in the 1950's and by 1989 there were 23 specialty and 51 sub-specialty boards in the USA.

Associated with this period is a loss of understanding by medical practitioners of the values of the society that they serve. Consequently, physicians have lost the ability to make moral and value decisions for their patients (Pellegrino, 1976; Callahan, 1980). This has had important implications for the way physicians perceive the subjects under observation (patients). They now became mechanical devices that may be adjusted and tuned as needed and typically of mechanismic systems, patients lose their individuality. Their wishes, fears and needs are superseded by physicians who analyze them in the laboratory (hospital) and even today, many physicians tell patients what is good for them and will not tolerate any deviance from advice.

Another subtle change of this period is that whereas both the community and the community of healers selected candidates for training as healers in earlier times, any person with ability could now apply for and be accepted for training as physicians. The focus, as Vickers pointed out, now was on individual rights and ability, and no cognizance was taken of whether the candidate may suitably fulfill the needs of society. The kind of individuals that became physicians changed. No prizes are given at the end of training for candidates who best understand their intricate relationship with patients or society, instead, those best able to satisfy the educational system win out.

---

[8]It was also the start of industrial man, the ultimate individualist. The interaction of individual wants with technological ability leads to the creation of a positive feedback mechanism and is part of the health care problem.

The introduction of machinery made mass production of medicines possible. These were now made and manufactured by businesses, bound by business interests and ethics, and the traditional chemist in time became no more than a distributor of drugs. As such they lost their status as professionals, which by definition they no longer are. Most pharmaceutical companies are driven by the need to show a profit on their investments (Taber, 1995). This has important ethical and moral implications. The success of a drug depends more on effective marketing than on research (Editorial, 1993). Widening the indications for the use of a drug often increases sales. Most pharmaceutical research is in areas such as lipid lowering drugs and psychiatric drugs, mainly because new discoveries in these areas are extremely lucrative.

Similarly, the hospital system developed to the extent that professional managers had to be found, which spawned an accompanying bureaucracy. Nurses became employees of this system, their first loyalty being to the hand that feeds them and patient interests today consequently became of secondary interest. Nurses now strike for better wages as common workers, the interests of the patient being secondary to their and the trade union's aims.

Until the 1930's, patients were themselves responsible for payment of their health care bills (Samuelson, 1993)[9]. Due to the increasing number of players, complexity and increasing costs, an increasing number of patients could no longer afford to pay in the traditional way, which lead to the introduction of medical insurance. The object of this was that patients would deposit funds with administrators as long as they were healthy and could then draw on this in times of need. Administrators negotiated payment with the different service providers, usually at a discounted tariff in return for guaranteed payment. This system rapidly grew to include virtually every member of society who could afford to join. Remuneration therefore no longer was an aspect of treatment to be considered and discussed between patient and physician, but became a negotiation between physician and administrator. Both service providers and patients became less aware of cost. To the latter, health care became a right in return for their insurance contribution. Administrators are essentially business people and their aim is profitability. This is reflected in the way in which patient funds are administered. In South Africa for example, and probably many other countries of the world, the relationship between administrator and physician rapidly declined to one of hostility and mistrust. The reason is that both are competing for a limited resource, namely health care funding.

---

[9] In 1925, one day's hospitalisation at the Massachusetts General Hospital cost $3 and was paid by patients out of pocket. By 1972, it cost $200 and only 12% of patients could pay out of pocket (Knowles, 1973).

The advent of medical insurance had another important effect. There was a time when patients would select a physician because of a good reputation as a clinician, or for being affordable, or easily available. Medical insurance however draws no distinction between different abilities and capabilities, all physicians are remunerated according to the same scale. Hence, it is a system that reinforces protection of the weak from the strong and tolerates inefficiency, and in addition, it removes from the system any form of competition between physicians, which, in the past, had contributed to cost containment.

Lastly, modern technology increased the life expectancy of the population. People want to live longer, but the longer they live the more likely they are to develop chronic illnesses. Modern society can no longer afford to care for the ageing population it had helped create. Furthermore, modern methods of birth control destabilized the birth arm of the birth-death balance in populations.

Information era

We are now in the transition to the information era (Toffler, 1990;[10]Ackoff, 1981). The body of knowledge available in even a single discipline like medicine is mind-boggling. It is also growing at an exponential rate and much of this knowledge is relevant for only a limited period of time. The challenge of this era will be the dissemination and constructive use of knowledge. In terms of the discussion so far, a solution to this problem is a learning organization. In other words, the solution lies in individuals starting to interact in formal human activity groups, sharing information and skills. There will be a survival advantage to those groups that can adapt and learn in a rapidly changing modern environment in a co-evolutionary manner. Those individuals who hope to go it alone will, like the boy facing the leaking dyke, find themselves with all their fingers and toes plugging holes with new ones forming all the time.

Worldview

> *"Every known human society is thought to rest on some set of largely tacit, basic assumptions about who we are, what kind of universe we live in, and what ultimately is important to us".* (Kriel, 1996)

What are the assumptions and mind maps that are fundamental to most thinking about the health care system? These may be divided arbitrarily into

---

[10]According to Toffler, people get power through the control of force (violence or threat of violence), money or knowledge. We are now entering the era where knowledge will mean power.

the mind maps about the health care system on the one hand, and of the physician on the other.

The worldview of health

The term "health" is frequently used in matters of a medical nature. We speak and write of health care, community health, tropical health, health certificates, health farms, health foods, and so on. The term is also used to denote certain organizations such as the National Health Service, the World Health Organization and Health Maintenance Organizations. But what does it mean?

The Concise Oxford Dictionary defines health as:

> *health* (n): **1** a state of being well in body or mind. **2** a person's mental or physical condition. **3** soundness. **4** a toast drunk in someone's honor.

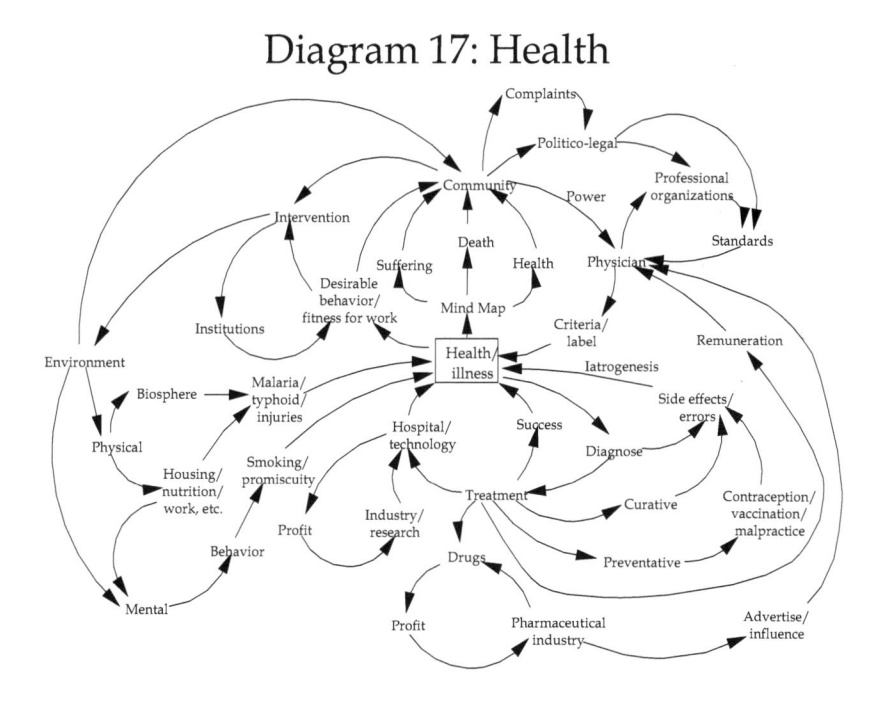

Diagram 17: Health

The latter two meanings are clearly of no relevance to the discussion, and the former two sufficiently vague to allow a large amount of latitude in understanding. And yet, when researching or planning, we assume that everybody know and are in agreement with what we have to say about health and health related issues. The term has become so submerged in our web of knowledge that we no longer question our understanding of it. But one is left with the suspicion that the concept "health" may be much more complex than the usually anticipated meaning. To test this hypothesis, the current worldview of health and its historic development is traced using System Dynamics modeling (see **diagram 17**). Ivan Illich's *Medical Nemesis: The Expropriation of Health* (1976) served as the main source of information for constructing the model.

Society, in response to a social need, transfers the power to determine what passes for "health" to the health care system in general, and physicians, as its representatives, in particular. In this way the health care system acquires the right to set the criteria for, and label the different causes of illness and health. It includes inter alia: What is considered to be illness, who is ill or healthy, who will be treated and in what way, and so on. These criteria and the processes that result from them feed forward to reinforce or alter the mental idea that society forms of illness and health. The model of "health" consists not only of the perception of what "health" is, or ought to be, but also the way that society experiences suffering and death, two conditions that are inseparably linked to health. Hence, in the first instance, the image is the result of the *interaction* between society and their agents, namely physicians.

The modern view of man as a machine is a product of the technological era. According to this view, specifications of normality may be determined scientifically, and any deviation from the so determined criteria constitutes abnormality. To physicians is therefore ceded the power to determine who is fit to do what kinds of work or for military service, who is to be admitted to hospital, mental institutions, etc. The way that a society classifies people determines the eventual functioning of that society, as well as the ways that society will attempt to alter its environment in order to conform to the classification. It also determines the form of the institutions that society will create for caring for the aged, the infirm, and the disadvantaged. According to this view, modern man therefore is a finely tuned instrument and any deviation from the norm (which may affect its ability to contribute to technological society) must be readjusted either by the health care system, or by the institutions created by society on their instructions.

The idea that suffering is an inevitable part of human life is central to most ancient and many modern cultures. As a result of our ability to remove pain by the use of modern technology, modern man has lost the ability to deal with suffering, not only individually, but also collectively. Pain is now considered to be unnatural and must be removed at all cost by the agents of society (physicians). In addition, the standards for survival imply that death before a statistically determined mean is unnatural. Hence, the health care system must prevent death at all cost and a failure to do so indicates a mistake on the part of the system. Furthermore, dying of an injury or disease is considered to be abnormal, the machine is meant to survive until it comes to a halt as a result of advanced age.

It may be true that the modern worldview of health resulted from the actions of the health care system and its members, but at the same time, society sanctions its continuation by insisting that the system carry on in its present form. Ordinarily, this would not present a problem, but for the fact that society can no longer afford the present system.

In the physician driven health care system, physicians diagnose and treat what they determine to be illness. To remove pain and prevent death, sophisticated apparatus are required that, because of their cost, is concentrated in hospitals, of which the purpose becomes to cure. Therefore, a high quality of "health" becomes associated with high technology hospital based care, and health in turn becomes merely a commodity that may be bought or sold.

It is accepted today that many of the treatments given by physicians either do very little to change the health status of patients, or might even harm them. Furthermore, such treatments often have side effects, which may require further treatment. Even diagnostic interventions may cause harm, either by itself, or by incorrectly diagnosing illness when not present, resulting in incorrect or inappropriate treatment. Illich calls these illnesses caused by physician intervention *iatrogenesis*. But the problem goes even deeper. The health care system, by screening the population, determines who *may* become ill in time and treats such cases prophylactically by vaccination, etc. For example, by prescribing contraception, pregnancy, a natural event, may be prevented. People who are *healthy* may become ill as a result of complications caused by preventative interventions.

Industries that supply the drugs and technology to cater to the needs of the health care system are profit driven, hence the more of their products consumed, the better they are off. They operate by canvassing the support of physicians as the prescribers of their products. This may be done by advertising, or many other creative ways to influence decision-making. Decision-making determines criteria and therefore the whole balance of the concept of "health". In addition, physician decision-making is also influenced by the remuneration they receive for their work.

Physicians form professional societies that inter alia determine the standards according to which they label illness. These societies are sanctioned politico-legally, but the politico-legal system may bypass the societies to set alternative standards by law if so desired. This route is usually followed when the community becomes unhappy with the present functioning of the system.

The communal environment consists of mental (internal) and physical (external) components. The former expresses itself through human behavior, some of which may result in illness, such as smoking, promiscuity, etc. The health care system may identify such behavior and declare it undesirable, which may lead to attempts by the community to alter behavior through laws, fines, etc. The physical environment consists of housing, the availability of water and a sewerage system, the work environment, etc., and what shall be called the biosphere. By the latter is understood those components of the environment with which we are in daily contact, such as soil, bacteria, insects, the weather system and all its components, etc. Both the physical environment and biosphere may be the cause of illness and therefore are frequently targeted for intervention. In fact, it has been shown that better housing, sanitation and nutrition improves "health" to a larger degree than direct intervention by the health care system. It is becoming clear that Western style health care does very little to prolong the lives of people suffering from congenital defects, diabetes, injuries, etc., but it is very efficient for improving their quality of life. In other words, in general, modern health care does little to prolong life, but it does make it possible for more people to live out their lives in a better way.

When society, on the recommendation of the health care system, intervenes in the environment, changes are made that in turn affect communal life. Hence, the health care system, by its recommendations, indirectly has a powerful influence on the interaction between environment and mankind.

On the basis of a System Dynamics model of health, it would be fair to draw a number of important conclusions.

1. Understanding the term "health" as the well-being of body or mind is simplistic and unsatisfactory.
2. The mind map that society holds of "health" is a complex constantly evolving concept resulting from numerous ongoing interactions. It has a history that may be studied, and a future that cannot be predicted.
3. Precise knowledge of our understanding of the term "health" is vital for scientific communication and also for health care planning. It lends itself in particular to intervention by the systems approach.
4. One may postulate that altering the mind map that society and physicians have of "health" may prove to be more rewarding in restoring the health care system to health than currents attempts to manage process. In fact, based on the system dynamics model, such interventions may prove to be counter productive and in the long term may do more harm than good.

5. Blaming the medical profession for the current ill health of health care systems has no meaning. It was caused by the <u>interaction</u> between society and the health care system and the solution lies in managing this interaction.

Associated with the worldview of health are the following historic relics:

- Medicine is a *calling* (a vocation (Allen, 1992)). Today, the university as the representative of society selects those candidates considered to be most suitable for the profession. Whether the selection process is suitable for the purpose of modern society is debatable, since the criteria used are based upon intellectual achievement and socio-economic ability, in other words the trappings of the technological era. The question arises whether medical practitioners trained by the educational system are suitably equipped to deal with the modern health care system in which they will find themselves. More so, are they the physicians that society needs?

  The concept of a calling prohibits physicians to act in any way that will harm their clients, which therefore means that they may not withhold their expertise (strike), etc. This restriction is enshrined in law in many countries.
- Training takes place by way of an apprenticeship. This is still true of modern medicine and in particular the surgical disciplines, but the basic primary care training more accurately reflects the ideals of the technological era with an emphasis on scientific method.
- In primitive societies the secrets of the medicine men were guarded. This is still true today where the knowledge of medicine is shrouded in unpronounceable Latin terms (Toffler, 1990). This reinforces the image of the professional.
- Medical practitioners are initiated into society during the taking of the Hippocratic oath. This ceremony takes place in the presence of members of the community and once this is completed the community confers on them the status of professionals.
- Medical practitioners form societies closed to laity, just like their earlier ancestors.
- The empirical knowledge base of modern medicine is based upon Cartesian determinism. This implies:

  a) A linear causality model.
  b) A mechanismic model of the human body and health care process.

  Furthermore, it implies a worldview of illness as the result of a malfunction in a piece of equipment and a disassociation with the spiritual side of illness.

- Patients have come to expect that many treatments imply hospitalization (Illich, 1976).
- The ability of patients to acquire information about their bodies and illness effortlessly, together with technological improvements have created health care wants that are often in opposition to needs.

This, the image that society has of health, describes a facet of the behavior of society as a system, hence it may be conceptualized as a regulator in terms of the health care system.

The physician

- Many physicians and patients still believe that most of medical diagnosis and treatment is *intuitive*. Although the medical student is trained within a scientific paradigm, when in practice, this knowledge is often ignored and decisions made intuitively "in the old way". Such decisions are then motivated as being "in my experience", which is arbitrary and untested and in a sense resembles ancient shamanism.
- Physicians are still afforded a special position in society, a legacy of the time when they were assumed to have mystical powers. As a result, they have a special relationship of *trust* with patients and the communities that they serve. Vickers showed that trust is an important regulator of stability in a human activity system. This relationship is coming under increasing strain in health care systems.
- Physicians are *professionals* and therefore presumed to be experts who know everything and who are always in charge (linear causality). Associated is the assumption that all professionals have the same amount of knowledge and skills (one is like the other). Furthermore, society has an image of how physicians should act professionally (bedside manner).
- Originally, patients interacted with physicians only. More complex societies meant more complex health care systems with the involvement of hospitals, nurses and pharmacists. Historically, physicians were in charge of and directed treatments. However, today the interaction has become complex to the extent that the concept of a physician in charge has little meaning. Interestingly enough, the legal profession still labors under the ancient mental model of medical responsibility.
- In the information age, the key will be knowledge and access to knowledge. For this to happen, aligned self-control is desirable.

This worldview of the patient-physician system has lead to some unresolved tensions, mostly as a result of a changing environment to which the worldview has not adapted.

- There is a tension between the intuitive, mystic approach and the empirical, scientific, specialized, high technology approach. This is

essentially a tension between the ancient shamanistic approach and Newtonian physics (precision and knowledge).
- There is a tension between a worldview of health care as a holistic communal problem and a focus on illness as an individual entity (reductionism).
- There is an opposition between the belief in the medical community that their profession is a science and the reality that much of the profession is borrowed from its environment.
- An increase in knowledge has lead to the necessity of specialization and super-specialization that has lead to an alienation from the patient. The reason is that the community of physicians has not been able to make the transition to a social system that is sharing a common worldview.
- There is a tension between a view of medicine as an ethical profession and the intrusion of business and business ethics on the other hand. This is the same tension that exists between commercialization and any other profession[11]. Business is about satisfying customer demands and hence the customer is always right. In terms of the definition of a professional, the professions cannot be businesses because of the inherent incompatibility in performance criteria.
- The result of the tensions is that the medical profession is faced with a total collapse of their ethical base and an inability to rectify it (a village commons situation). There is also an increased alienation between physicians as representatives of their community and patients (Levey and Hesse, 1985).
- There is alienation between physicians amongst themselves and in particular between generalists and specialists.
- There is a tension between the medical needs and wants of patients Saward, 1973).
- The concept of physicians as professionals is in conflict with what they can deliver. By definition, the physician is a professional[12] expert who has been taught from a body of knowledge to assist patients in restoring a perceived physical or mental dysfunction (Allen, 1992). This means in effect that physicians put to the disposal of their patients (clients), special knowledge and skills in return for remuneration. To do so, tools will be used from the larger medical system to assist them in diagnosis and treatment.

In summary, in this chapter it was shown how the health care system grew from a simple one-on-one interaction into a complex human activity system, but with an underlying worldview of illness and process based upon

---

[11] J.P. Strümpfer: personal communication.
[12] A professional: a person belonging to a *vocation* or *calling*. An expert: someone having special *knowledge* or *skill* in a subject. Accordingly, the definition of a professional will be: a person who is called, and has special knowledge or skill.

simplistic linear thinking. This is therefore the dilemma of medicine as it is being practiced today. It can be illustrated most starkly in its simplest interaction, namely the patient-physician interaction. Furthermore, in terms of this proposition, this is the level where intervention could potentially have the biggest and most beneficial effect upon the system as a whole. In the next chapter, this interaction will be analyzed against the argument developed until now.

Chapter 8: The Patient-Physician System

The patient-physician interaction is the first and simplest interaction of the health care system. The purpose of this interaction is to decide upon a course of action to solve a patient's problem. Although nominally only two people are involved in the interaction, it is one of high complexity. The beliefs and expectations that patients and physicians have significantly increase the number of permutations to be considered in decision-making. Added to this is the complexity of the illness processes itself (the knowledge component) since the efficiency with which knowledge available to the system is utilized is a function of the efficiency of the processes and interactions in the system. The decisions that physicians and patients make ultimately determine how the health care system will be utilized to address the patient's problem. The eventual measure of this is the cost to the system. Therefore, the interaction between patient and physician sets into motion a train of events that consists of the interaction between a number of players in a complex human activity system. It is proposed that the system can be improved, with an ultimate saving in cost, by improving the decision-making process. The latter may be improved by testing and changing the beliefs of patients and physicians and by the improved utilization of available knowledge in the system.

The discussion will be based upon the assumption that:

- Health care is in the first instance the responsibility of patients. They may be assisted to achieve this by physicians.
- The consultation process is influenced by the worldviews of illness and of physicians as professionals. Patients and physicians have their own versions of these worldviews.
- Diagnosis ought to be a learning cycle, rather than the current linear process.
- The diagnostic cycle is an analytical process based upon the manipulation of knowledge and experience. It suffers from the same constraints of knowledge as other scientific disciplines.
- Treatment is influenced by the decision-making process as well as the concept of control assumed.

The patient-physician system

For the purpose of this text, the patient-physician system will be defined as a system where a person (patient) consults[1] a professional (physician) about a

---
[1] *Consult*: to seek information or advice.

perceived change in his/her physical or mental well-being, for the purpose of obtaining reassurance, or to have the change restored or altered to his/her satisfaction. The components of this system are:

- The patient
- Physician (family practitioners and specialists)
- Pharmacist
- Hospital system and
- Administrator

All of these are part of the larger health care system. In reality the patient-physician system cannot be seen in isolation, since it is affected by input from the larger health care system, which in turn is influenced and affected by the larger social system. The boundary selected here is therefore arbitrary in order to create a snapshot in time for analysis and discussion.

What is understood by the term "health care"? An often quoted definition is: *the complete physical and mental well-being of all humans and not merely the absence of disease* (World Health Organization definition (Ulrich, 1994b; Agnew et al. 1965). This definition is vague and consequently does not stand up to rigorous examination. According to the Concise Oxford Dictionary (Allen, 1992), health is a state of being well in body or mind, and care a thing to be done or seen to. Health care could therefore be a state of well-being of body and mind that must be done or seen to. Another more comprehensive definition, is Henrik Blum's: *health is a state of being in which the individual does the best with the capacities he has, and acts in ways that maximize his capacities* (Ulrich, 1994b). This definition emphasizes purpose and personal responsibility and will be the operative definition in this text.

Who must see to it? In terms of a social system model and Blum's definition, it is the responsibility of individuals themselves to seek the well-being of their own bodies and minds[2]. To achieve this they may be assisted by health care workers such as physicians and also by other elements in the individual's social environment (politicians, civil servants, and so on). The focus of this study is the interaction with the physician.

The fundamental interactions of the system (illustrated in **diagram 18**) are:

- Physicians make special knowledge and skills available to patients in return for remuneration (Kass, 1983).

---

[2]The difference between patients' rights as opposed to their responsibility is often confused (De Wet, 1991). There is also a difference between equity and equality (Ackoff, 1981).

- Patients invest funds during periods of health with administrators who manage the funds and reimburse relevant parts of the health care system on behalf of the patient in times of illness. In return they are allowed a management fee (Teisberg and Porter, 1994).
- Specialists have knowledge and skills of a higher order than the family practitioner (McWhinney, 1989)[3].
- Hospitals make facilities and equipment available to physicians, which enable them to practice their knowledge and skills.
- Pharmacists stock medication, which physicians prescribe to patients.
- Specialists, hospitals and pharmacists are remunerated for their service by health fund administrators.

Diagram 18: The Patient-physician System

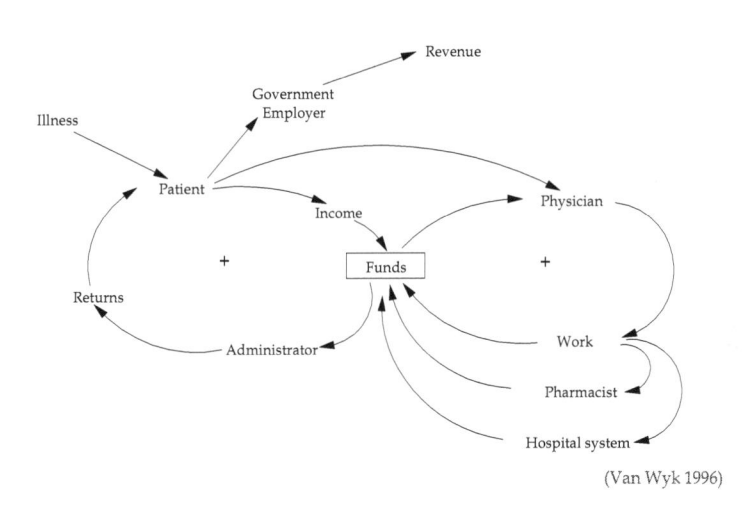

(Van Wyk 1996)

In terms of process, two interactions can be identified as problematic in the present system. Firstly, there has been a breakdown in communication between physicians and administrators, each of who see each the other as deadly enemies. The reason for this is competition for health care funding, a limited resource. Physicians respond to the threat by attacking the patient. This can be done through over servicing, unnecessary procedures, padding of accounts, and so on, in other words, by increasing the volume of work done. Administrators are powerless to prevent this and have to charge ever-increasing contributions from patients to cover their escalating costs. This is a

---

[3] The implication of this in the current health care system is that specialists are used by family practitioners as a resource. This kind of approach is inefficient in terms of a learning organisation model.

village commons situation caused by a limited resource, namely health care funds.

The problem is that at the same time the physician's actions also fuel the hospital and pharmaceutical side of the system (unintentionally). This accelerates the funding loop, which is a reinforcing loop until patients find themselves in a situation where they can no longer afford health care. They then put pressure on their representatives in government or their employers who feel obliged to intervene. The depletion of health care funding also puts pressure on government and company revenue. Companies who cannot control the health care costs of their employees lose their competitive edge and cannot compete in world markets (Levinsky, 1984). The actions of physicians therefore affect not only the health care system directly, but other associated systems indirectly as well. The only way to prevent these two reinforcing loops from running together, is by implementing a shared idea of the patient-physician system, in other words by self-aligned participation by the patient, physician and administrator in the health care system.

Diagram 19: The Patient Physician Interaction

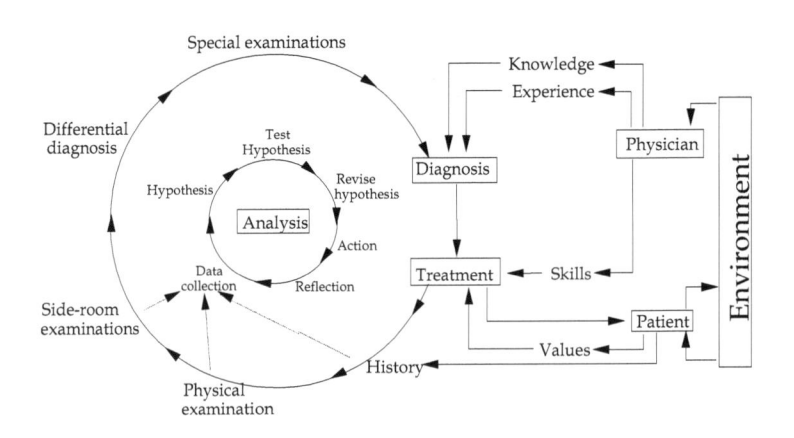

Secondly, there has been a breakdown in communication between family practitioners (FP) and specialists. This leads to double prescribing, the repeating of expensive tests, lost time, and so on, actions that also fuel the cost spiral in the system as a whole. This happens because the diagnostic-treatment system has to be cycled through twice instead of once. It creates a problem of inefficiency in the use of knowledge that will be discussed later.

The consultation system

The consultation system is the axis around which the patient-physician interaction revolves (see **diagram 19**). Patients access the system to resolve their illnesses. The purpose of physicians as professionals is to bring their knowledge and experience to bear on the problem in an analytical way, in order to find a reasonable explanation for the problem (diagnosis). They use their skills to put their theories to test by way of treatment. Once the problem has been satisfactorily resolved, both patient and physician return to their respective environments and the interaction is concluded. In terms of this interaction, physicians are managers of illness.

The patient-physician interaction basically involves three processes.

   i. The consultation, which is the interaction between patient and physician.
   ii. The diagnostic process.
   iii. Treatment. (Diagnosis and treatment are traditionally considered to be the responsibility of the physician).

The consultation

This involves the patient, the physician and the patient's illness. The wants and needs of both patients and physicians contribute significantly to the complexity and outcome of decision-making. These are often not made explicit and are usually difficult to quantify. These images will be the topic of discussion in the next two subsections.

The patient

A person receiving, or registered to receive medical treatment (Allen, 1992)

Both the illness (or problem) and the experience of it is a function of the environment in which patients live. The patient's problem and the expected experience of the consultation can be the result of an expectation, a want, or a need. Illness will be discussed separately for the sake of clarity and not because it can be separated from the consultation. Illness in this discussion will be assumed to be an expression of the patient's wants or needs.

   a) Expectations

Expectations are shaped by the personality of patients and their previous experience of similar problem situations (what they have learnt). These expectations lead to mind maps of health care that determine the demands that patients make on the health care system.

Patients have a perception or expectation (image) of their problem and its possible resolution. Such images come from personal experience as well as the reported experience of other people. They may have experience of someone they know who has suffered from a similar complaint before. Such an experience has a powerful influence on expectations about their own problem situation and its possible resolution.

The influence of the 'lay press' in shaping perceptions about illness and the medical profession cannot be underestimated (De Wet, 1991:9). Often patients have read about a specific condition such as prostatic cancer and by the do-it-yourself questionnaire attached, found symptoms that they imagine being the result of this condition. The fear of cancer is then the reason for the consultation. Images are often clouded by the fact that reports in the lay press frequently are an incorrect representation or misrepresentation of reality. The question of the value system and the subsequent responsibility of the printed press are an important systems question in this regard.

Cultural expectations play an important role in forming an image of disease, particularly in a culturally diverse country such as for example South Africa. For example, young black men sometimes complain of impotence. Further questioning then reveals that they are unable to produce multiple performances in one night. To the mind trained in medicine within our Western cultural framework this is nonsensical, but within a framework of African culture, it is not (Mbiti, 1971). The diversity of cultural attitude creates problems in the medical system, as we know it. Firstly, we are not trained to deal with multi-culturality, but more importantly, our medical system as we know it is the product of our Western cultural heritage (Vickers, 1969). This means that physicians trained in this paradigm are unable to deal with this kind of complexity in terms of the environment within which it has meaning.

The question then is should this system be changed to include these expectations and if so, how? Can we attempt to integrate African, Eastern and Western systems into a single medical community, as we know it? For example, it is important in African culture to prove your ability to procreate. Unmarried patients will therefore often be referred for help. The problem now is that current health care funding does not support this kind of treatment. More so, it does not support this treatment in unmarried couples. The patient can now have the necessary treatment in a private capacity, but very few can afford it. The reason such treatment is not supported, is that it is considered to be a want and therefore not necessary. However, from a cultural point of view it is important that the patient should be helped, because they may find themselves ineligible for marriage or even relationships in their own cultural environment. This leads to stress and other related problems. There is of course an ethical question as well. Should we contribute to the population problem that the world suffers from and also possibly to that of homeless children. Cultural expectations therefore introduce great complexity into the consultation.

The cultural problem has another aspect. In Europe, homeopathy, osteopathy and aromatherapy are popular alternative treatments and of course in the east, treatments such as acupuncture, etc. These "doctors" can now practice legally in this country and may solicit referrals from medical colleagues. The dilemma is that by far the majority of these treatments that have been tested in terms of the Western scientific tradition have failed that test. For example, phytotherapy (herbal treatment) for benign enlargement of the prostate is as good as no treatment at all (Fitzpatrick et al. 1991). Furthermore, most physicians have experience of cases treated by alternative medicine that went horribly wrong. These schools, rightfully so, point to their success in treating cases in which Western medicine has failed patients, the dilemma being: why did the treatment work? It may be that the reason is the well-known placebo effect, or just simply an alteration of lifestyle to a healthier one. The fundamental difference between Western style medicine and alternative treatments is in the rigor of diagnosis, the latter being more representative of the ancient paradigm. Therefore, the question may not be why alternative treatments work, but can traditional healers diagnose accurately? If not, they will contribute to the cost problem through deferred treatment. The point is that such healers could potentially be accommodated in the health care system, but that would entail a change of thinking about the system.

Finally, the importance of culture is the fact that it represents the larger social system within which patients and their problem ought to be seen and which includes both patients and the medical system. It is widely accepted in the medical profession that medical treatment, primary health care, high technology medicine, etc., contribute very little towards a healthy population. The biggest gain comes from adjusting the social system (Illich, 1976). By creating employment, a person can afford a proper home, food, sewerage, and so on, and this indirectly has an impact on health (Cowley, 1993).

Patients have expectations of the physician that they consult, in other words, an image of physicians, as they perceive them. The image of learned professions is based upon an assumption of knowledge and skill.

> "Patients expect to benefit from medical care. They consult a doctor because of his skill. They trust him to exercise his knowledge and skill to the best of his ability, and they assume that he will take all reasonable steps to ensure a favorable outcome" (McIntyre and Popper, 1983).

Physicians derive their authority from their assumed knowledge and skill, the belief being based upon a linear causality concept, in other words, it assumes that physicians are in full control of the situation. It has been shown earlier that control by an individual is only feasible in a simple deterministic system, which medicine is not. This issue will be raised again in the discussion of the image that physicians have of themselves. The question is what knowledge and skills do physicians have to justify this image?

Another assumption, based upon the same model, is that physicians as professionals all have an equal amount of knowledge and skill. Therefore, it does not matter who you consult the outcome will invariably be the same. This is a mistaken belief and may have potentially serious consequences. Furthermore, it leads to the inefficient use of resources and therefore has cost implications. It may be that this assumption is fundamental to the fact that patients select physicians on grounds other than knowledge and skill.

Table 6: Selection of Family Practitioners	
Good with children	17%
House calls and available after hours	14%
Friendly	11%
Has enough time for patient	9%
Knows what he is talking about	9%
Trust in his judgment	8%
Accurate diagnosis	6%
Interested in the patient	6%
Listens to your problems	6%
Reasonable rates	6%
Makes me feel comfortable	3%
Refers when necessary	3%

The image or expectation that patients have of physicians influences their selection of service provider. For example, patients tend to consult physicians on the basis of a word-of-mouth advice, either by a layperson (friend or acquaintance), or another physician (referring physician). They will select specific physicians because of their "good bedside manner" or "because they are wonderful with children", but rarely because they are known to be competent or well qualified. I have often been told myself that patients expected an older physician, since "specialists are usually older and more experienced". Such an image may lead patients to question the validity of an opinion, because of a presumed lack of experience.

A market research conducted for Sherag (Anonymous, 1992) showed that patients selected practitioners for the reasons indicated in **table 6**. The interpretation of the results depends on whether the right questions were asked, how they were asked, and so on. However, in spite of such reservations, conclusions can be drawn from the data. The table suggests that the selection of physicians is based, as suggested above, on imponderables such as good with children, available after hours, etc., and there appears to be an implicit assumption that all physicians are knowledgeable and skilful. On the other hand, how do patients know if the diagnosis has been accurate and the standard of care sufficient, other than measured by their own expectations of the outcome (Teisberg and Porter, 1994)? Even medical practitioners have difficulty in judging the competence of colleagues in disciplines different from their own.

Patients have an expectation of what treatment to expect. For example, they may believe that there is a cure available for the common cold, although medical science has not managed to secure one yet. They may come with a suitcase in hand, in case they will be admitted for treatment, because they expect hospital treatment or surgery. The problem is that sometimes physicians are influenced in their decision-making by patient expectations. This has cost implications.

Patients (at least some of them!) have an expectation of an eventual remuneration for the consultation. In early history patients expected to pay directly and promptly for the service rendered, but the modern position is that patients contribute to medical insurance and expect this source to take care of any financial implications of the visit. This leads to an expectation that the service is a right and free and that they can expect their expectations of the visit to be met (Anonymous, 1991). This is a fundamental problem and weakness in any "free" medical care system such as NHS. Many patients are unhappy if their complaint is not covered by insurance, the blame usually being placed on the physician who is considered to be the cause and culprit.

b) The illness

Of fundamental importance is the worldview (image) of illness within which the consultation takes place. In the present health care paradigm, illness is viewed in a reductionist way, in other words a linear cause and effect model. The emphasis is therefore on the perceived cause and the eradication of the cause, the process seen as the one necessarily following the other. A competing worldview is a systemic view, where the illness is seen in terms of the environment in which it happened and within a system dynamics model. Such an approach would be more in keeping with the complexity of physiological processes and their disturbance in the form of illnesses.

The deprivation model of illness is a linear model that assumes that illness can be removed by removing deprivation and poverty (Charlton, 1994). The redistribution of wealth and income is seen as sufficient to remove illness as a problem from society. This model has been used in approaches to health care both by systems thinkers (Anonymous, 1994b) and non-systems thinkers (Leutwyler, 1995).

In a complex causality model with multiple feedback loops, there are many factors that are necessary and that interact to cause an illness, even though a single symptom may be prominent and the focus of concern. Differences in illnesses are only in the complexity (number of co-producers) of the interactions leading to illness (product). Even a simple problem such as a cut may have a number of co-producers. Why was the knife not in its normal place? What interaction with the parent led the child to ignore the warning not to play with the knife, etc. In the case of a cancer, the complexity is such that we have a very limited understanding of why the growth occurs. This discussion has an important point. A comprehensive treatment will attempt to address as many of the co-producers of the illness as possible, even though the immediate focus may be on the problem itself. If this is not possible, there should be an awareness of the fact that the problem is not dealt with in total and in many cases not at all. The focus then will be on the symptom of the illness, which in effect is the current Western illness paradigm.

Because of their belief in a simple linear cause-effect model of illness, both patients and physicians believe that if the "right" treatment is prescribed, the illness will inevitably disappear. In reality, because of the complexity involved, physicians rely on the probability that an illness will be cured given that a treatment that is known to help is prescribed. Furthermore, treatments themselves interfere with complex biological systems, and although believed otherwise, cannot target only one interaction in such a system. Hence, all treatments have unwanted side effects. Fortunately, usually these effects are minimal and go unnoticed, but sometimes they present as complications of the treatment, such as the drug side effects, which most people experience sooner or later.

The prevailing concept of causality has an important influence on medical research and consequently medical knowledge. It has an even more important influence on the belief of physicians that they are in control of the diagnosis and treatment. A linear concept of causality is the cornerstone of the managed care medical audit system.

The consultation may be the result of the wants or needs of patients. For example, a patient may want to have a small upturned nose. Having it is not a necessity, however the current health care system makes it possible for this want to be satisfied. Modern technology largely focuses on addressing health wants, for example the current shift towards keyhole (laparoscopic) surgery. Patients do not want incision scars and modern equipment makes that possible through improved technology. However, there is no proof that such technology is cost effective, in other words wants in this case lead to increased cost. The problem is therefore: patient wants → technological discoveries to support wants → increased work → increased cost.

On the other hand, the patient may suffer from tuberculosis or malnutrition, the treatment of which is a need that has to be satisfied. The distinction between wants and needs is not always easily discernible.

The illness itself may be the result of the patient's environment. An example is an industrial accident or industrial illness, such as pneumoconiosis. Tuberculosis and meningitis are conditions associated with crowding and therefore poor socio-economic conditions. Post-traumatic stress disorder is likely to be more frequent in times of war and civil violence. Attention to the social environment therefore has an important role in reducing illnesses caused by the environment, which in turn may have a positive effect on cost.

The historical background of a society as part of its social environment can be a co-producer of illness. For example, the Afrikaner in South Africa has an inordinately high incidence of familial hypercholesterolenemia and consequently coronary heart disease. This is the result of intermarriage, in this case in its widest sense. The fact is that a genealogical investigation quickly reveals that the Afrikaner people originate from a very small genetic pool.

Some illnesses are self-inflicted. The common example is smoking, which is now generally accepted as being dangerous to health. In spite of this, a surprising number of people still persist with it. Another example is AIDS, which can potentially be eradicated by simple social measures. A study amongst young people in a number of first world countries indicated that the majority of them are aware of this illness and measures for protection against it. And yet, only a small percentage is actually heeding this advice (Anonymous, 1994a). Self-inflicted illness as a problem affects cost.

Some patients have illness built into their life scripts[4]. To them the health care system is an emotional support system. Mind maps are therefore influenced by a personal attitude to illness. These are the patients that will often move from physician to physician if they are not satisfied that the advice that they are given fits the model of what they expect. The problem is that in these cases psychological intervention to remove the script will often leave them with no script at all and create a new even more complex problem. It is also true that the current system of payment and support makes it highly undesirable for these patients to play out their scripts, yet at the same time the structure of it allows them to do so. In terms of causality, the personal

---

[4]A script is an ongoing program developed in early childhood under parental influence, which directs the individual's behaviour in the most important aspects of his life (Berne, 1987).

script leads to illness, which reinforces the script through a reinforcing loop. The problem is that the illness at the same time affects cost loops.

Sometimes, the perception of symptoms is quite obvious, a broken arm is bent in an unnatural angle or a strange lump is in an unusual place. Many symptoms however, are based purely upon the subjective appreciation of patients themselves. How does one understand pain or impotence? We try vainly to measure such complaints, but in the end they have a metaphysical component that cannot be encapsulated into a scientific truth or law. This is the problem of image formation and the transfer of such images to other people.

People diagnosed as being ill by the physician occupy a special role in society namely the illness role. This role accords them with certain obligations and privileges. For example, they are exempted from social obligations and are not held responsible for their incapacity (McWhinney, 1989). The way that patients experience illness and accept their role is a personal one determined by individual personality. Once they accept the role, they are obliged to seek professional help and also to make every effort to get better. Some patients will fail to consult, even when they have a serious problem and others will consult for minor problems that could have been solved with self-care. The reason for this is that the environment of patients often shapes their decisions. For example, failure to consult may be caused by unemployment caused by illness, religious beliefs, lower socio-economic class, and so on.

In summary, patients have a complex worldview in place that is the product of the interaction between their environment and their personality. It creates expectations about the consultation and the outcome of their treatment, and therefore affects the system in terms of cost. Changing this worldview could markedly influence the system, which could indirectly have a beneficial affect on the system as a whole and therefore cost. Important aspects of this worldview are:

- The concept of illness and health care.
- The image of the physician as professional. This includes the ideas of authority, control and knowledge associated with this position.
- The complexity that the worldview adds to the consultation process.
- The expectations (demands) of the health care system that the worldview creates.

Another way of looking at the wants-needs dilemma is in terms of purpose or function. Needs have to be satisfied to ensure survival and physicians are the means for achieving this. However, wants have an ethical component that questions the desirability of many patient expectations. Therefore, a worldview that has the ability to address purpose has the potential to influence the system.

The physician

A person legally qualified to practice medicine (Allen, 1992).

As in the case of the patients, physicians are the products of their environment. Their mind map of the interaction is created in a similar fashion to that of patients and they also have expectations, wants, and needs that is part of the consultation. These images add substantially to the complexity of the interaction.

Possibly the most important part of the model is the image that physicians have of themselves as professionals. Physicians tend to take on the image that the interaction which society demands. It may be that in some cases physicians take on the role they *assume* society wants of them, for example surgeons may take on the role of a "cutter". Take note here that it is not what society *ought* to get from them, in other words what they were taught during their training. It is a peculiar fact that once physicians qualify, they ignore much of what they have been taught. They tend to resort to practicing the craft in a piecemeal way based upon personal perceptions (images) of what they ought to do. The most fascinating aspect of this change is the way that they motivate their actions. This leads to a perception of medicine as being "a medley of science, magic, and inspirational guesswork" (Boulding, 1987) when the profession is observed from the outside. The problem is not with the process, but in the way that physicians as professionals act.

A study is quoted in New Scientist (Kingman, 1994), where researchers wanted to test a specific treatment for adult respiratory distress syndrome. At the start of the study it was found that less than 40% of physicians used the standard protocol for ventilation. The question is why do physicians have this propensity for altering treatment to fit their perception of what it should be, as opposed to the protocol that they ought to follow? Or put differently, why do they no longer follow the accepted protocol? This is an essential weakness of the professional as individual decision maker.

The image that physicians hold of themselves has another more serious weakness built into it. This is the assumption that medical students once qualified have acquired the complete body of knowledge of the profession (or at least knows 50% of everything depending on university regulations). Society sanctions this belief by granting them a legal license to practice their craft by virtue of their registration with medical council. They are now presumed to be professionals and "authorities" and the latter is someone society assumes does not err (McIntyre and Popper, 1983).

The stage is now set for a tragic situation, namely the fact that the worldview of an "authority" includes the assumption that they can seldom be wrong. Physicians often make mistakes, but to uphold the image of authority these mistakes can never be admitted. From here it is a short step to a belief that professionals do not make mistakes at all and integrating this into the personal image of a physician. Furthermore, the whole concept of learning by experience becomes meaningless unless there is a conscious effort to identify mistakes, analyze them and develop a strategy to avoid them in future. McIntyre and Popper make the point that the ultimate authority is our teachers in the halls of learning and that they have the biggest incentive of all not to be wrong. The deceit even starts with the examination of our students, which is a system that punishes students for mistakes and rewards them for hiding their ignorance. From a systemic point of view, a further complication is the fact that the admission of mistakes by the medical profession will not only seriously undermine the fragile image that society have of the professional, but may also put members at risk for legal action, a growing industry in most parts of the world (Claassen and Verschoor, 1992).

Many suggested changes to the health care system threaten to erode the position of the physician as a professional with a subsequent loss of authority and control and, more importantly, status. It is possible that if this happens, the type of candidate who has selected medicine as a profession until now will no longer be willing to enter the profession. In other words, those candidates who put a high premium on individual freedom of movement and choice will be lost to the profession. This will have a profound effect on the kind of physician that will eventually be in the system, and in time may cause unforeseen change to the system.

Physicians also bring their own personalities into the consultation. This includes their own cultural heritage and image of illness. For example, physicians who grew up in the East may be more inclined to have a holistic approach to the problems of their patients. Also, physicians with a high pain threshold are less likely to prescribe strong narcotics to patients. The fears and insecurities of physicians, as well as their own illnesses also become part of the consultation. For example, narcotic addiction or schizophrenia may adversely affect the interaction. To uphold the image of the professional, there is a code of silence in medicine that prohibits any physician from commenting on the competence of a colleague. There is a danger in this. Furthermore, the cultural heritage of physicians may create ethical problems in decision-making. For example, a Catholic physician could have difficulty with abortion and contraception as treatment options (Gillon, 1985).

Finally, physicians have an implicit assumption that they will be remunerated for their work, be it indirectly by an employer or directly by patients or their medical insurance. This is based upon a relationship of trust with patients. The trust is eroded when medical insurance claims are defaulted upon.

In summary, physicians also partake in the process of consultation with an enormously complex image of illness and health care in place that is the product of their environment as well as the health care system of which they are part. This includes the important self-image of a professional with its assumptions about knowledge and effectiveness. The worldview of physicians of illness and medical process therefore also has an influence on decision-making and cost.

Any intervention that has the ability to alter the worldview of patients and physicians could have a profound influence upon health care delivery and therefore cost. Aligned self-control in a social system model of organization is an example of such an intervention.

The remarks about purposeful behavior of patients apply to physicians as well.

The diagnostic system

The purpose of the diagnostic process is to collect information and manipulate knowledge. If the diagnostic system is not used properly as an inquiring system, knowledge will not be used efficiently and decision-making will result in inefficiency and increased cost. This paper aims to show that the diagnostic process is not functioning properly at present and that this, as a component of the patient-physician interaction, contributes to the problematique of health care. Efforts to increase the efficient use of knowledge in medical decision-making may contribute to a more efficient system that is more cost effective. Traditional diagnosis is a linear process, but it becomes more valuable when reconceptualised as a circular process of inquiry, or learning system. When health care interactions are functioning properly, the flow of knowledge becomes more efficient.

Diagnosis

The first step of a consultation is when patients explain their observed symptoms or concern to a physician (they pose a question). Physicians then start an empirical process during which information is gathered (inquiry). This they do by questioning patients about the problem, its previous history and their background, in other words, they try to form an understanding of both patients and their illnesses in terms of their environment.

The process whereby information is gathered continues during the physical examination. Physicians will use all their senses, their eyes for observation, touch for palpation, ears for percussion and auscultation and smell for examination and side-room examinations. From the data collected a problem list (differential diagnosis) is constructed and possibilities tested by way of special examinations such as laboratory tests, X-rays and endoscopy. The physician is then ready to make a diagnosis (state a hypothesis) and test it by way of treatment (this is fundamentally the cycle of inquiry of traditional science, see **diagram 20**). Traditionally, if the treatment is successful the process ends and the physician is reimbursed (Pistorius and Pistorius, 1986).

Diagram 20: The Diagnostic Cycle

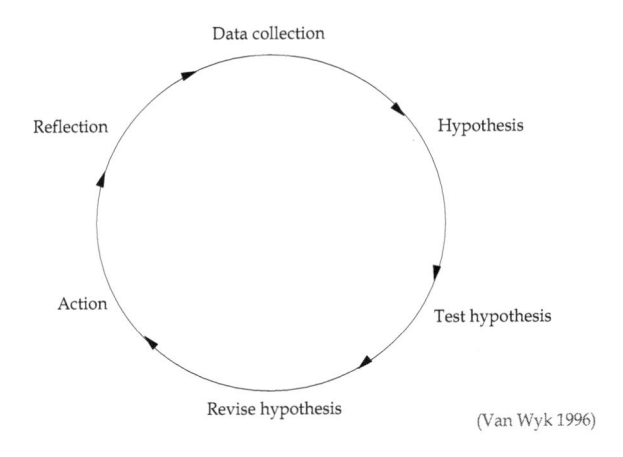

Data collection
Reflection
Hypothesis
Action
Test hypothesis
Revise hypothesis

(Van Wyk 1996)

If one looks at the diagnostic system taught to medical students, the essential observation is that of a linear system (Pistorius and Pistorius, 1986; Chamberlain and Ogilvie, 1974). The dilemma with such a system is that it results in the practice of cookbook medicine. The formula is followed to the letter and like a cake, fortunately it usually results in a favorable result. However, it is a static approach and as such not very efficient. Looking at the classical diagnostic system again, one can differentiate three stages:

i. Observation and the collection of information.
ii. Speculation based upon available knowledge and experience.
iii. Action (treatment).

Another way to look at this system is to alter it to its logical form, which is a *circular* process (see **diagram 21**).

Diagram 21: Medical Diagnosis as a Learning Cycle

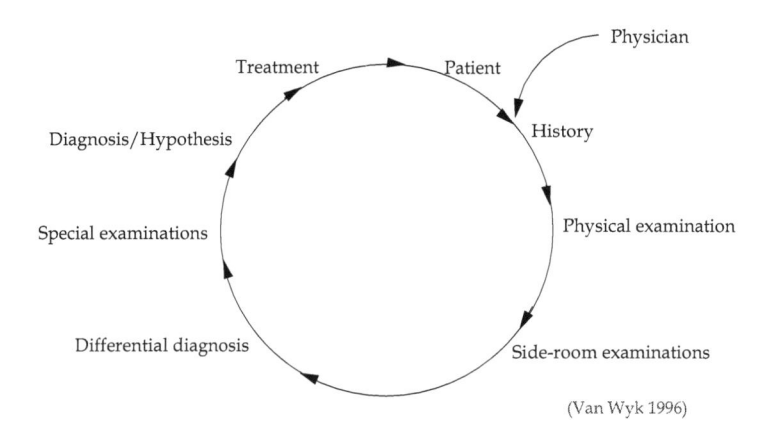

```
                    Treatment → Patient      ← Physician
      Diagnosis/Hypothesis              History
      Special examinations              Physical examination
      Differential diagnosis            Side-room examinations
```

(Van Wyk 1996)

The cycle starts when patients consult a physician (professional) about a change they have detected in their physical or mental status. The physician then gathers more information by taking a case history and by examining the patient. This data is integrated with the physician's own available knowledge and after reflection a provisional diagnosis (hypothesis) is postulated. This diagnosis is tested by the use of special examinations and treatment is then instituted on the basis of the diagnosis (thesis). The important last step is to observe the effect of treatment for future reference. Did it work? Why did it work or not work? How can I use this information in a similar situation the next time? Should the treatment be adjusted or changed to improve the result? What did I learn? The end point for patients is the satisfactory solution or resolution of their problems.

The diagnostic cycle therefore in reality ought to be a learning cycle and the process of diagnosis a learning system. There are two important components of the diagnostic cycle:

i. Experience. Learning can only take place in a system where reflection takes place, therefore a circular system.
ii. Knowledge. A poverty of knowledge has a detrimental effect on the efficiency of the system as a whole.

If we now take another look at the diagnostic cycle a frequent problem is seen. Many physicians tend to *bypass* the full cycle and form their hypothesis (diagnosis) based on a brief history alone (see **diagram 22**). The physical examination is either abbreviated, or often left out altogether. Such an approach leads to diagnoses based on a shoestring budget and cannot be reconciled with either good scientific method or proper medical process. The reasons for this approach are multifactorial, some being; a perceived need to accommodate a large number of patients within a short period of time (for monetary reasons, due to a shortage of physicians, and so on), a belief in the physician's own perception that the process is unnecessary as a result of his experience, and so forth. Some physicians solve the poverty of information problem by resorting to further investigations in the hope that any shortcomings in their approach will show up in the tests and can be rectified as a result. Furthermore, they assume that testing will protect them from possible litigation (Claassen and Verschoor, 1992). This is an expensive, inefficient solution. It is also a system lacking knowledge. It may be that this error occurs as a result of the tension between traditional intuitive medicine and modern "scientific" medicine, in other words the persistence of an archaic image.

Diagram 22: Abbreviated Diagnosis

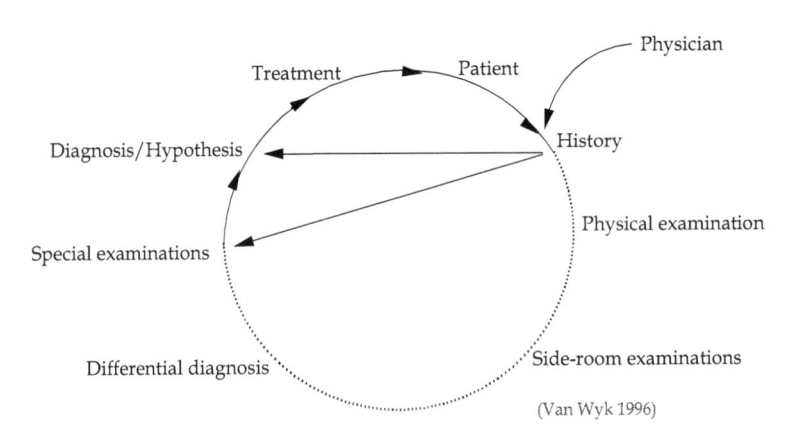

(Van Wyk 1996)

The problem becomes magnified when the incorrect hypothesis is acted upon, that is treatment is prescribed. In most cases the outcome is relatively innocuous, but when surgery is advised it can have a more serious outcome. In 1976 specialists in Los Angeles County embarked on a go-slow action during which only emergency procedures were performed. Over a period of five weeks the rate of surgery dropped by 60%. At the same time the mortality rates in the area dropped to the lowest level in five years, which promptly returned to "normal" when the strike ended (Cowley, 1993). The question arises, do physicians contribute significantly to the death rate and how? One reason could be the use of a poorly functioning diagnostic system.

A further problem is that a poorly functioning diagnostic system cannot operate properly as a learning system. By not integrating a complete set of information, very little learning takes place and furthermore possibly may lead to incorrect learning. A vicious cycle is then created when such incorrect data becomes part of the physician's knowledge system, the end result being poor medical care, which in turn influences the cost of health care delivery.

It is the submission of this paper that the outcome of the treatment ought to be observed and reflection should then take place about the process and outcome. This phase of reflection is vital for the learning process and for experience to take place. Within the traditional method, experience comes by repetition, almost by a process of conditioning, whereas in the suggested model experience is part of a process of conscious learning and the diagnostic system therefore becomes a learning system.

Knowledge

In terms of the diagnostic cycle, one has to ask what is medical knowledge and how is it acquired? Traditionally, medical students are given a prescribed list of reading usually one book for each discipline, which is augmented with lectures and practical case studies. If at the end of their prescribed number of years they can convince their lecturers that they absorbed more than the minimum amount of information required, they are deemed to know enough about medicine to practice their craft. This approach gives rise to two absurdities. Firstly, the medical curriculum is known by students to be *"one per cent inspiration and ninety-nine per cent perspiration"* (TA Edison quoted in (Cohen and Cohen, 1971)[5]. In other words, it lends itself to the memorization of a large body of data. But in the process, little attempt is made to teach in addition to this a formal approach for retrieving the information in a logical way (Weed, 1968). The result is that the majority of physicians have a cookbook approach to their craft. You compare your data to that accumulated in your brain, find a match and apply a formula that is supposed to work. The educational system reinforces the idea of the physician as authority, by contributing to the assumption that physicians have complete knowledge.

Secondly, the idea that learning the contents of an extremely limited number of texts will confer a broad and sufficient knowledge of the profession is ludicrous. A paper published in Scientific American showed that if all the medical journals abstracted in the Medline bibliographic database for one

---

[5]The original quotation was about genius, the remark is adapted for this text.

year were to be stacked on top of each other, it would form a pile one and a half times as high as the Washington Monument, which is about 500 feet high. This data is captured annually on 960 CD ROM's (Stix, 1994). More importantly, 50% of the data will be obsolete within five years of publication (Ackoff, 1991). The amount of data absorbed by the average medical student pales into insignificance in comparison with this. To cap it all, there is no mechanism taught to these students to continue with self study, hence subsequently the majority of physicians will make no more than a rudimentary effort to acquaint themselves with the knowledge explosion in their discipline. The question then is, how much <u>do</u> physicians know (Brook, 1994)? The answer is partly determined by the academic system of which they were trainees.

In some medical schools in the USA it is no longer necessary to cover all the disciplines in the medical field. For example, in 17% of all medical schools no formal lectures are given in Urology and in the remaining 83% the number of lectures in this discipline average 8 in the whole curriculum. This translates into a situation where 10 to 15% of graduating students have *never* been exposed to Urology (Benson, 1994). Approximately 3 to 5% of visits to generalists are for Urological complaints and 6% of acute hospital admissions are for problems related to this field. The question then is, how much do generalists know, how do they deal with these cases and how can they act as gatekeepers for specialist Urologists?

The knowledge explosion forced the profession into breaking up into specialized disciplines, which in turn are fragmenting even further. The problem is that many physicians now know more about less. This lead to an alienation from the patient. There is no reason to expect this trend to slow down and within this scenario, one has to question the viability of generalists in the future (Editorial, 1995), or probably more accurately, their present role. This is the fundamental weakness in the managed care concept of the generalist as gatekeeper (Anonymous, 1994b; Schwartz and Aaron, 1984; Teisberg and Porter, 1994). The question is; how can a person with an insufficient knowledge base be expected to determine when a more specialized service is needed?

The cost for treating an incorrectly referred or treated case is a serious problem. From a systems point of view a system with a poorly functioning gatekeeping design is doomed to become even more expensive in the long term. The challenge is to organize the large body of expertise into a coherent and well functioning whole. From this point of view, the generalist's role becomes extremely important, but only if it is redefined. It is a fact, that the practice of high-quality medicine produces fewer complications, better long-term results and subsequently lower cost (Teisberg and Porter, 1994; Milstein et al. 1989). The role of the family practitioner ought to become that of securing and accessing such high-quality care. In terms of the discussion until now, the challenge is to alter the referral system into a learning system based upon the principles of a learning organization.

The problem with a poverty of knowledge has a further important point. It is difficult if not impossible to form a proper hypothesis without a proper body of data (both knowledge and experience) which to refer to. Galileo would never have been able to discover the relativity theory in his time and neither would Einstein have if he were Galileo's contemporary. In the framework of medical diagnosis it is therefore difficult if not impossible to make a proper diagnosis without a sufficient database. Under such circumstances the diagnosis can be no more than Boulding's inspired guesswork (Boulding, 1987).

The difficulty of the patient-physician interaction during a medical consultation has been described before. But there are further additions to the complexity of the diagnostic process.

Many consultations are for complaints that are difficult, or in many cases impossible, to interpret or quantify. Physicians only have the assurance of patients that they do indeed have a headache and they have to rely on the appreciation of patients that the headache is severe. This situation may be complicated by intricate psychosocial interactions that may contribute to it, such as an unhappy marriage, a fear for cancer, and so on.

This intuitive problem that exists in the patient's experience, now has to be integrated with known medical knowledge. The problem with this knowledge is the epistemological question what do we know and how do we verify the accuracy of what we know? A major problem in medicine is the fact that up to 80% of treatments given to patients in good faith are untested for their ability to effectively solve the problem (Kingman, 1994).

The present situation is that medical knowledge is based upon fact nets (Eddy, 1990b), often with dubious privileged contingent truths at its base. Many of these truths are of historical origin and are being perpetuated from textbook to textbook. When examined more closely, they are often found to be incorrect and which causes whole fact nets to collapse. For example, Lowsley (1912) examined a small number of neonatal prostates in 1912 and from this data concluded that the adult prostate consists of six lobes. This is still quoted as being correct as late as 1970 (Hutch and Rambo, 1970), but in 1972 John McNeal (1972) published his findings of dissections of adult human prostates, which conclusively showed the model to be incorrect. This finding had a profound effect on modern research about the prostate, since the fact net supported by Lowsley's theory effectively had to be replaced.

Unfortunately, a very large part of medical knowledge is based upon such theories and needs urgent revision (Brook and Lohr, 1985).

Furthermore, many treatments have been in use for countless years. When originally introduced they were valid within their time frame, but within a newer enlarged knowledge base they are no longer so. However, since in many cases they do not cause any obvious harm, the profession is loath to re-evaluate and discard what is no longer appropriate (Anonymous, 1991). One such example is the dilatation and curettage (D&C), which is frequently performed in woman and which in modern medicine has very limited indications, since better diagnostic tools are available. Yet, it is still commonly performed (Kingman, 1994). Another such procedure is neonatal circumcision, which can very rarely be justified by current medical knowledge alone (Wallerstein, 1985). There is therefore a need to systematically re-evaluate the foundations of medicine and to substantially correct the errors that are present (Brook and Lohr, 1985).

It has been suggested that medicine as a profession is not a science, however there has in recent years been an effort to give the profession scientific legitimacy. There is a noticeable shift towards a logistic community of inquirers (Eddy, 1990a). In other words, more time and money is spent within the profession on basic research and the ability to publish (or perish) is based upon the reviews of appointed or elected experts. The problem then becomes the deficiencies of the logistic system. The number of publications secures the legitimacy of researchers in the community and this expertise in turn allows them to decide upon the merits of the publication of other contributions. This therefore becomes a self-perpetuating cycle.

Furthermore, there is a very heavy reliance on statistical methods to measure and interpret data. The aim of these methods is to serve as a measure of predictability. Predictability (or the probability that an event will occur) in turn depends on a reliance on predictable systems and therefore linear causality. It has been argued elsewhere that biological systems in general and health care systems in particular are non-linear (Goldberger et al. 1990). In addition, health care systems are social systems, which increase the complexity manifold. The measurement of human systems is an enormously complex problem and yet, today it is a prerequisite for medical publications.

The position then is are the right questions asked and are the conclusions drawn from them valid? The outcomes of medical interventions have potentially serious effects and the margin of error allowed is therefore very small. Who then guarantees the validity of medical research? The problem is solved by way of the community of experts (Feinstein, 1988; Eddy, 1990a), who answer such questions by agreement amongst themselves (Eddy, 1990b; Eddy, 1990a). The medical community granted these physicians this position and their work is used to serve as an example for others. How do we know that the community selected the right candidates and how do we know that their work is correct and ethical? The most important criterion at present appears to be the number of publications attached to an individual's name. There is a problem that the editors who choose the publication of texts are also a community that perpetuates itself. The danger of this is that important work may be denied publication whereas weaker papers are selected, because they are submitted by the right institutions or authors and are presented in an acceptable way. Furthermore, it is fascinating to see in medical literature papers where more than half of the quoted references are papers authored or co-authored by the writer (for example Labrie, 1993). They themselves therefore give themselves scientific legitimacy. The point is therefore that this approach is a flawed one and that there is a danger in accepting a community of experts as a model for the medical profession.

It is interesting to note that the pharmaceutical industry uses this reliance on the community of experts to promote their products to physicians. The way that this research is presented can profoundly influence the attitude and approach of physicians (Forrow et al. 1992; Naylor et al. 1992). If the data and conclusions are flawed, the communication is flawed and can potentially have serious effects. Products are introduced through the publications of selected experts. An underlying problem is the fact that by far the majority of these authors have had an incentive for publishing the data, either as a result of direct sponsorship, or indirectly by supporting the presentation of data at medical meetings that secures additional prestige, and so on.

Even if the data is presented accurately, the interpretation can be incorrect (Smith and Egger, 1994). Wiswell (1992) presented a lecture during which he concluded that there are strong indications for neonatal circumcision. A meta-analysis was done of studies indicating a link between non-circumcision and urinary tract infections in boys. The findings were that infection occurred in 1,38% of non-circumcised boys, as opposed to 0,11% of circumcised boys, a more than ten times higher incidence. The conclusion was that this would support the advisability of neonatal circumcision. Furthermore, according to the author, sexually transmitted diseases almost exclusively occur in non-circumcised men and can therefore be prevented by circumcision. There are a number of problems with this study.

- The implication is that to prevent 1 incident of urinary tract infection (a non-fatal condition) amongst 100 boys, 99 will have to be circumcised unnecessarily. The procedure is not free of complications.
- The conclusions are based upon a linear causality model. In terms of multiple causality a number of questions arise such as is the circumcision rite more frequently performed in higher socio-

economic classes, in other words are there other reasons that can explain the findings?
- Furthermore, only 1 - 4% of uncircumcised boys with colonization with uropathogens under the foreskin developed infections. This appears to indicate other co-producers.
- Wiswell asks the question whether uncircumcised boys have a higher rate of congenital malformations. It is not clear how neonatal circumcision after the fact will affect fetal development.
- The idea that circumcision prevents sexually transmitted diseases is emphatically wrong.

The problem is that this presentation at a prestigious meeting, contributes not only to fact nets, but also to the application of a dubious treatment on a large number of cases.

The traditional way of research in medicine is by way of randomized clinical trials. However, this approach suffers from a number of problems, such as the fact that they are time-consuming and expensive. Sample sizes are limited, there is difficulty in drawing conclusions about narrowly defined groups and they are usually performed under ideal circumstances (best physicians and best facilities)(Brook, 1994). The RAND Corporation recommended an alternative method, namely the synthesizing of the knowledge and experience of experts (Brook et al. 1986; Brook and Lohr, 1985). The immediate problem is who are the experts, how do we know they are experts, how do we know that the experts have correct knowledge, how do we know they will ask the right questions, what influences them into being part of the panel, who decides who the experts are, and so forth?

Medical research is based on a scientific model of control of the laboratory by the experimenter. In a highly complex environment, such as the patient-physician interaction, the experimenter has virtually no control over the experiment and its outcome. Any conclusion drawn from a clinical study has to be considered very carefully for its validity.

In conclusion, there is a dilemma about the scope of medical knowledge. The implication of this is that whatever knowledge is available ought to be used to the maximum effect, but with circumspection at the same time. Incorrect knowledge leads to incorrect decision-making and incorrect learning in terms of a learning system. This in turn has important implications for the delivery of quality health care. The community of physicians determines the scope of medical knowledge. This is a complex social system in its own right and the proposals in this study are equally valid when applied to this group.

On the other hand, the current paradigm is to install into medical students a database of information that is assumed to be complete, correct and sufficient for life. In terms of a learning system model, a method for retrieving relevant information and gaining experience from it is more important than a rigid body of knowledge. This discussion therefore suggests that the current system of medical education is no longer appropriate in a modern health care system. A system is needed that will lead to thinking about illness in terms of wholes, and the principles of a systems approach may be an appropriate candidate for such a methodology.

Diagram 23: The Traditional Gatekeeper System

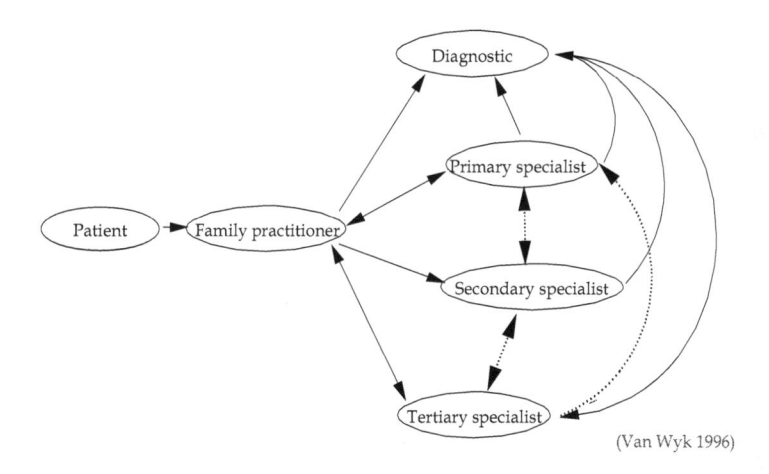

(Van Wyk 1996)

The specialist referral system

Specialist. *A person who is trained in a particular <u>branch</u> of a profession* (Allen, 1992), or: *a physician who devotes himself to a special class of diseases* (Agnew, 1965).

Additional access to the knowledge system in medicine can be gained by using the specialist referral system. This system (**diagram 23**) consists of:

- The primary specialties (pediatrics, internal medicine, gynecology, anesthesiology and otolaryngology). Most referrals are from family practitioners and self-referrals from patients.
- The secondary specialties (general surgery, reconstructive surgery, orthopedics, urology, gastro-enterology, cardiology, neurology, and so on). Most referrals are from family practitioners and other specialists.

- The tertiary specialties (high-technology disciplines such as cardio-thoracic surgery, neurosurgery, oncology, and so on and the super-specialties). Most referrals are from other specialists.
- The diagnostic specialties (radiology and pathology). Referrals are from family practitioners and all other specialists.

In terms of this structure, referrals to the diagnostic and primary specialties are almost exclusively from family practitioners and self-referrals. As the complexity of the discipline increases, more referrals come from other specialists. Any system that interferes with this system will affect the viability of the high-technology disciplines and also the delivery of services by them. The gatekeeper system used by managed care to control physician process and cost is such an intervention.

The purpose of the specialist physician is to make special knowledge and skills available to the patient or referring physician. In the traditional system, patients will consult the family practitioner, which will refer them to a specialist for a consultation or treatment. McWhinney (1989) understands a consultation to mean that a person who *may* be a specialist is consulted. The patient is at no time under the care of the consultant unless referred and the opinion of the consultant is not considered to be binding, in other words a recommended course of action may be ignored. Referral implies the transfer of responsibility, although this transfer is considered to be partial only. A study was done that showed that 97% of exchanges between family practitioners and specialists are referrals and only 3% consultations (Rakel, 1990). There is an underlying assumption that family practitioners are in control of the patient-physician system and that specialists are a resource that may be accessed by them (McWhinney, 1989).

The specialist referral system exhibits the following features:

- The family practitioner in the traditional system is the gatekeeper in charge of the patient-physician interaction (Coulter, 1992; Hillman et al. 1992). The gatekeeper concept is fundamental to all current models of change where control is implied and in particular in managed care and primary health care models (diagram 6). The assumption is that specialists are a major cause of the escalating expenses in the health care system, because they use expensive medication and are the main users of hospital care, which is a large contributor to the cost problem. Furthermore, it is assumed that keeping patients away from specialists will keep them away from hospital care and in this way there can be a major cost saving. In managed care systems, gatekeepers are rewarded in various ways (usually financially) for not referring patients, as an incentive to ensure compliance (Hillman et al. 1992).

In managed care systems specialists are discouraged from re-referring patients to other specialists. Patients are to be referred back to family practitioners that decide whether re-referral is necessary.

Gatekeeping is a cause of resentment to specialists. They feel that generalists withhold patients from them until their patients are in dire trouble, with a subsequent increase in the difficulty of problem solving and increased cost, which in turn is blamed on the specialist, with more gatekeeping, and so on. Furthermore, as generalists do more work that is traditionally assumed to belong to specialists, there are less referrals and a reduced income. Specialists then have to find ways of supporting their income, with more unnecessary procedures and treatments being performed, increased costs, more gatekeeping, and so forth. The gatekeeping concept therefore has a tendency to affect cost in a negative way. It has been suggested that gatekeeping eventually may only have a minimal effect on cost saving (Milstein et al. 1989).

On the other hand, there is a feeling amongst generalists that the traditional pupil-teacher relationship, which is the prevailing model in teaching hospitals, is perpetuated in the generalist-specialist interaction. This is a cause of resentment amongst generalists (Balint, 1986). Many consultants act towards family practitioners as if they have a higher standing, which inhibits communication and consequently the flow of information. This in turn leads to increased cost, which reinforces the specialists' perception and therefore the pupil-teacher relationship.

There is an underlying assumption that generalists have a broad knowledge and skill base that qualifies them to fulfill the gatekeeper function and which allows them to control the situation. In terms of a complex social system model and the discussion about knowledge, this assumption is a fallacy (Berwick, 1991).

The problem with a gatekeeping system is the following. Firstly, it is based upon a linear causality model, which has serious shortcomings in a complex system such as the health care system in terms of control. Secondly, it is a barrier to the efficient flow of knowledge, which in turn leads to inefficient practice and therefore increased cost. In terms of a social systems model, this concept has to be addressed in order to achieve aligned self-control. Such a system will have the potential to improve efficiency and therefore reduce cost.

- It is a misconception that specialists know more or is more skilful than generalists, the only difference between them is in the depth and width of knowledge (Rakel, 1990). This belief, combined with the gatekeeping concept, means that if specialists share their knowledge and skills with generalists, they are likely to lose more work, with a reduced income, and so on. This affects cost, which in turn leads to more gatekeeping. It is therefore a barrier to the free exchange of knowledge in the health care system. Furthermore, in countries such as South Africa, all specialists were originally trained as family practitioners. In principle, they have the same knowledge as family practitioners, their specialist training adding to the scope of it. This assumption is based on the idea that professionals have complete knowledge.

Only generalists have the necessary insight to select the appropriate specialist for a particular patient. The proper consultant is selected by the following criteria (Rakel, 1990), knowledge, skills, a personality compatible with the patient, availability and the ability to work well with the referring family practitioner. In practice the choice of specialist is based on functional rather than technical qualities, therefore some of the best qualified and competent specialist physicians often have the smallest practices.

A number of years ago, a person who only had a Standard 8 School Certificate was found to practice as a specialist pediatrician in South Africa. He had referrals from "fellow physicians" for four years before his lack of expertise was detected. The implications and ramifications of this are mind-boggling. For one, no one (colleagues, hospitals, medical insurers and patients) ever asked to see proof of his qualifications or registration with the medical council. It would appear that there is an extraordinary trust in the medical profession and even amongst colleagues. The point is that a system that rewards an intuitive approach in preference to knowledge and skill can only be an inefficient system. Furthermore, available knowledge and skills in such systems are not used to their optimal potential.

- Reasons for referral or consultation are the following (Dixon, quoted in Rakel, 1990), for diagnosis (7,8% of referrals), management, diagnosis and management, patient request and for confirmation of a diagnosis or plan of management. On average, 2,7% (1 - 5,4%) of family practitioner consultations are referred. The highest referral rate is for women between 15 to 44 years. Most of the referrals are for conditions affecting the neurological system and sense organs, followed by the genito-urinary system. Accordingly, most referrals are to neurologists, ophthalmologists, otolaryngologists, gynecologists and urologists. These findings may reflect the demographic pattern of referrals.

Fewer cases are referred in a FFS system (3,19%), than a managed care one (4,46%). The question then arises are cases not referred because family practitioners are competent and have no need for consultation, or because they are incompetent and do not diagnose problems that ought to be referred (Rakel, 1990)? A further cause may be that it is more lucrative to treat patients in a FFS system, in other words family practitioners may do more than they ought to.

In summary, the referral process has a potentially large influence on patient care (Grant and Dixon, 1987) and therefore indirectly cost. The current system is based upon a worldview that is the result of the historic development of the health care system. This view is an obstruction to the flow of knowledge and is therefore inefficient. The dilemma can be resolved if the prevailing view is tested and the format of the specialist system changed. The solution therefore lies in transforming the referral system into an efficiently functioning complex human activity system. Such a system ought to be a learning system.

Testing

A differential diagnosis is frequently tested by way of special investigations. The two most commonly performed groups of examination are:

- Endoscopy; and
- Laboratory tests.

a) Endoscopy

Endoscopy became very popular in recent years. This is the result of an improvement in lens systems, fiber optics and better lights sources. It therefore becomes possible to observe parts of the human body from the inside such as with gastroscopy (the stomach), cystoscopy (the bladder), arthroscopy (joints), and so on. The problem is that the interpretation of what endoscopists observe is highly subjective. Not only will the finding be influenced if they do the examination blinded to the background history, but also if repeated in the same patient on a number of occasions. As a result of this it is a notoriously difficult procedure to teach. The possible error rate becomes compounded by the perception that physicians have of the problem. For example, they may ignore significant findings in a patient that they perceive to be a hypochondriac (error of the first kind), or diagnose an abnormality when it does not exist (error of the second kind).

The assumptions of the teacher may become part of the mental model of the student and if incorrect the error is passed on and probably magnified from generation to generation. In both instances, action based upon the interpretation of data not only has potentially serious consequences for the patient, but also affects the cost of the health care system in total. Endoscopy therefore is a relatively simple examination, but the interpretation is enormously complex and fraught with error.

b) Laboratory testing

The problem for the pathologist is similar to that of the endoscopist. Studies have shown significant variations in interpretation between qualified observers and also in the same observer on repeated evaluation of the same specimen. The possible error may have grave consequences. For example, for suspected carcinoma of the testicle the organ is explored surgically. During the procedure the vascular supply is interrupted to prevent spread of the suspected tumor along this route and a biopsy is then taken of the suspicious area. The pathologist will then examine the specimen in the theatre and the organ will be removed depending on his finding. I have experience of such a case where the pathologist reported a benign lesion and two days later realized that he had made an error. In this particular case this did not affect the prognosis, but in another case the outcome may have been grave.

Another area of error is sample collection. There is a very specific way that urine samples should be collected to yield accurate results (Kunin, 1987). Many patients will report that it has been done incorrectly when asked how their specimens were collected. This may be as a result of ignorance of the technician doing the collection, lack of interest, etc. This can lead to error, the possibility of which has to be included in any decision-making process. Furthermore, in the laboratory situation the usual errors of measurement may occur. Was the processing of the specimen correct, was the equipment functioning properly (has it been properly calibrated), has the technician been properly trained in using the equipment, has the reading been taken correctly, etc. Some of the mistakes are errors of process, in other words occur when the testing protocol was not been followed accurately.

Human error needs to be considered. Has the specimen been correctly labeled and handled. For example, after-hours urine samples must be refrigerated until they can be transferred to the laboratory. The person doing the collection may have neglected to do so and may hide the fact to escape censure. Specimens may be switched. The reality is that even in medical systems errors occur, but due to the seriousness of such error the margin allowed for error ought to approach zero.

The significance of error becomes serious if the indication for the tests is wrong (if the wrong question was asked). Blind faith in the ability of testing is a source of error, because tests are a guide and must be understood to be such. Furthermore, the use of tests to compensate for a lean diagnostic cycle could potentially lead to serious error.

The laboratory testing system is therefore a complex system on its own with many interactions that contribute to the successful completion of a test.

However, the possibility that errors in such a complex interaction may have occurred must always be born in mind. Furthermore, due to the seriousness of errors, workers in such a system ought to share a strong ethical worldview. The problem of diagnostic testing is that of laboratory process, which is similar to testing in all scientific disciplines.

In summary, diagnostic testing is a complex process. The possibility that errors may have occurred always has to be considered in the decision-making process, since such errors could have serious consequences if acted upon. The reliance on special examinations to compensate for an abbreviated diagnostic cycle (insufficient process) is therefore a high-risk strategy. Therefore, special examinations contribute to knowledge about the problem, but are not in themselves a safe substitute.

The problem is that of the accurate verification of knowledge, which is similar to that of any other scientific discipline. The implication is that physicians ought to have knowledge of the process of inquiry to improve their decision-making ability.

Treatment

The successful resolution of a patient's problem depends upon how the decision to treat was made, and secondly, how well the decision is implemented in practice.

Decision-making

The decision about the appropriate course of action to solve the patient's problem is based upon the integration of the result of the diagnostic cycle (empirical component) with the expectations and wants of patient and physician (intuitive component).

The decision to treat and the treatment recommended is often influenced by patients, their perception of the problem, their expectations of treatment and the way that these perceptions are transmitted to the physician (McNeil et al. 1982). Preferences for treatment are not based upon scientific data but rather pre-existing beliefs. For example, often when a conservative approach is recommended patients will ask if they will not be getting a prescription, because many patients associate a prescription with good treatment. Or they may insist on an antibiotic for a cold, or flu (and get it), because it is "usually given" even though there is no medical reason to do so. Physicians fear that they will get a reputation as poor professionals should they not oblige. Some patients insist on surgery even though it may not be necessary. The whole practice of reconstructive surgery is an example, where the most important reason for treatment usually is vanity. The problem therefore is a wants-needs dilemma. Physicians may take on the role that they sense patients expect of them, which in turn leads them to negate the protocols that they have learnt, with a subsequent effect on quality of treatment and cost.

There is a wide variation in comparable treatments administered by different physicians (Wennberg et al. 1989; Brook and Lohr, 1985; Teisberg and Porter, 1994; Eddy, 1990c). Factors contributing to this are training, experience, knowledge, attitude, and so forth. Decisions are made within the perspective that an individual has of the problem (Tversky and Kahneman, 1981). If there is a chance that there will be a gain from a decision, decision taking will avoid risk, but if there is a perceived chance of loss, decision-making involves risk taking. This means in the medical context that if it appears certain that a specific diagnosis is correct, physicians will not take the risk of selecting an unlikely hypothesis. But if patients are likely to have an adverse experience, they will be prepared to take risks. Furthermore, decisions are taken not logically (even in people trained in logic), but based upon biases that are part of the mind maps that people, including physicians, have (Tversky and Kahneman, 1974). This is why many medical decisions are based upon intuitive grounds rather than more logical, well-motivated reasoning.

There is also a large variation in decision-making amongst individual physicians. Observers looking at the same problem will disagree with each other 10 to 50% of the time. They will also change their minds 8 to 37% of the time when confronted with the same problem again (Eddy, 1990c). The implication is that many treatment decisions are wrong, both in the sense of a mistaken perception of the facts, and because they are not in the patient's best interest. Such errors are usually not deliberate.

The approach and attitude of physicians to the problem influence the treatment. For example, many surgeons believe that any condition is potentially curable surgically. They would be more inclined to recommend surgery as opposed to physicians who are more conservatively inclined. Two fascinating examples of the dilemma created for patients when they are given conflicting opinions about treatment by different disciplines were published in Fortune magazine (Alexander, 1993; Grove, 1996).

Another important factor in decision-making is the influence of the environment. Important players here are business (the pharmaceutical industry and managed health care) and the state. In both the managed care and state health systems there is an incentive to control the physician. Many physicians probably join these institutions in the mistaken belief that if they are salaried they will not be influenced by the financial incentives referred to earlier. However, they exchange this comfort for control. For example, in some institutions in South Africa, heart transplants are no longer allowed. This creates a number of dilemmas. Firstly, there is the ethical dilemma that physicians face knowing that there is a treatment available that may help or even save patients. The question now arises; who makes the decision for withholding treatment, and more importantly who takes the responsibility? The problem of rationing is also one that is important in managed care. Why is the decision made to ration heart transplants? Should other expensive treatments then also be rationed and if so which ones? Who decides which treatments are acceptable and which ones are not, and how does one know that the decision is the right one? Human lives are dependent on these decisions. This has become an ethical question of a village commons type and Vickers is correct in believing that time is running out and sooner or later difficult decisions will *have* to be made. Those decisions and the responsibility for them will have to be of a socio-political nature.

The fundamental difference between state control and managed care are the beneficiaries of the system. In the former the state, and therefore society, stands to benefit, but in the latter, although some schemes are ostensibly of a non-profit kind, the industry benefits. For example, medical aid administrators receive approximate 10% of turnover as commission. For example, in 1994 in South Africa this amounted to R16 million. In the case of Medicross, SA Druggists control the company who in turn is part of the Malbak group. They therefore effectively sell the medical insurance that forces patients to attend their system, in which they control physicians who prescribe the drugs that they manufacture. The director of this company stated in public that the object of Medicross is to support those patients unable to afford full medical aid, but with a sufficient income not to be state patients (Benningfield, 1995). The fact is that they have not built any clinic other than in areas with a high density of traditional medical aid patients. The motive therefore is profit, mostly indirectly, as shown.

The potential remuneration involved impacts on whether treatment will be given and which treatment will be preferred (Engelhardt and Rie, 1988). A drug, finasteride, was launched as an alternative to the surgical removal of the benign prostate gland in men. It is widely accepted that prostatectomy represents approximately 20% of the surgical caseload of urologists and this procedure therefore represents a significant part of their income. As was to be expected, the drug was received rather frostily by the urological community, something that the manufacturing company found difficult to understand. Treatment, and in particular surgical treatment, is more likely to be recommended should the physician be in a difficult financial position. This is likely to happen more often around the time that income tax payments are made, and if there is an incentive such as a shareholding in the clinic in which the procedure will take place.

But it is not only the physician's remuneration that is involved in the decision. The whole health care system has an impact. For example, I treated a case in a private hospital and two weeks after discharge saw the patient again with a minor problem that needed readmission. The private hospital would not admit him again, because his medical insurance was exhausted. In other words, once the purse is empty they have no further moral obligation to attend to a patient in need, even though the treatment process has not been completed. The problem could not be treated at home, because there is no adequate infrastructure to do so safely (an environmental problem). The state hospital would admit him only as a fully paying private patient if a private practicing physician (myself) continues the treatment. Alternatively, he had to be admitted as a state subsidized patient, provided his treatment is taken over by the government employed physicians (a control and decision-making problem). The fact that the attending physician felt morally and ethically obliged to continue treatment and was prepared to do so on a *pro deo* basis was not considered to be significant in the process.

The pharmaceutical industry has a large and unaddressed interest in remuneration in health care. During 1994, 30% of medical insurance payments in South Africa were for medicines. If the drugs and other items that are part of hospital bills are included as well, the figure is 50%. This amounted to an amount of R8 billion. It is a fact that these companies are businesses with traditional directors who report to shareholders whose main interest in the company, in turn, is their dividend (Garattini, 1997). The purpose of the directors is therefore to ensure as large a dividend as possible for their shareholders. The value question of whether this should be done at the expense of sick people is an unanswered one. It is true that no new antibiotic has been discovered during the past twenty years (Bylinski, 1994). The reason is that the largest part of research is spent on the development of cardiac drugs, which is an extremely lucrative market. It is possible to cure many more people with more effective antibiotics than with cardiac drugs, but with less profit. The same is true for the research into medication for AIDS. The chance of finding a cure for this disease from a biological point of view is slim. However, the company that does so will have discovered the pot of gold at the end of the rainbow. Again, the value question of whether society benefits from this is unanswered.

There is a perception in the medical community that health care is either essentially free (government medicine), or purely a business transaction. If the latter position is to be accepted, the rules of decision-making are no longer governed by traditional ethics, but by the profit motive. It is easy to come to such a belief, seen against the background of supporting health structures, which are motivated by profit.

There is data that suggests that decision-making ought to involve patients. The attitude and values of patients are the key to selecting the correct treatment for a particular case (Wennberg, 1990; De Wet, 1991), since patients will have to live the consequence of the treatment. An important point is that at the moment we do not really know what patient preferences are for treatment. At present these preferences are decided by physicians who may have a preference for specific treatments that differ from that of patients. Wennberg in his paper concludes that the answers to health care problems will be found when physicians (and patients) come up with new ideas, in other words when they start interacting efficiently as a complex human activity system.

In conclusion then, the decision to treat, and the specific treatment recommended, is usually assumed to be a simple empirical decision based purely on medical indications. However, decision-making in reality is influenced by patient wants, needs and expectations, physician wants, needs and expectations, and the influence upon both of the other components of the health care system. In other words, the decision-making process can be influenced to suit the wants of patients, physicians and business interests in the health care system. This has serious implications in terms of the cost crisis in health care, and measures to correct this problem therefore have the potential to have a beneficial influence. It is proposed that the use of systems thinking may increase an awareness of how the decision to treat is made, which in turn may influence the consultation system.

Implementation

The decision to treat and the specific treatment recommended again opens up a number of complex interactions.

There is an implicit belief amongst physicians that they are in full control of the consultation (Marwick, 1992). In terms of a complex human activity system, they probably control no more than half of the interaction at best. A large part of the consultation is made up of observer (physician) bias and the expectations of the patient (client). The rest being the scientific part or inquiry that may be controlled. The control of complex interactions is virtually impossible, and the consultative process is an example of such a process.

Equally, although they usually believe the contrary, physicians control only a small part of the treatment process (Rutstein et al. 1976; De Wet, 1991). Berwick (1991) described some of the processes involved in an open-heart operation. A successful outcome will depend on.

- Whether the diagnosis is correct. This depends on whether the diagnostic cycle was followed correctly, which depends on the physician's knowledge and experience, the patient's co-operation, a properly functioning diagnostic process, and so on.

- Whether the surgeon is competent. This depends on training (which depends on the educational system), experience (which depends on the number of similar cases performed), continuous education and whether active learning has taken place.
- Whether the blood bank cross-matched bloods correctly and has the blood in the right place at the right time. This, in effect, is a laboratory system with all the attendant interactions.
- Whether the blood gas analysis machine works properly and the technician is trained to use it properly. This in turn depends on the manufacturing system that has produced the equipment and the competence of the technician, which in turn depends on training.
- Whether the suturing and other equipment has been manufactured without any defects. This depends on a well functioning manufacturing and delivery system.
- Whether the nursing staff is competent to recover the patient. This depends on their training and whether the hospital has the necessary equipment available and these are functioning properly for them to perform the task.
- Whether the anesthetic machine has been connected properly, has been calibrated properly and is functioning properly, in other words similar interactions to the other equipment.
- Whether the medication from the pharmacy has been labeled correctly. This in turn depends on a properly functioning dispensary system.
- Whether the instrument tray has been sterilized and packed properly, etc. This depends on a functioning sterilizing system, in other words the whole process that instruments has to go through to be sterilized, including intervening human interactions.

The outcome is therefore dependent on a large number of highly complex interactions that includes the purposeful interaction of a number of related components and systems. In this highly complex interaction, the surgeon as an individual can control only a relatively minor part directly.

In the end, treatment is an implementation problem. In other words, it has to do with those actions necessary to ensure that plans made to resolve the problem situation (illness) during decision-making (diagnosis) are executed as prescribed. Traditionally, treatment is implemented in a similar fashion to all planning be it corporate or otherwise, and as a result, suffer from the same problems. Most planners and managers are aware of the fact that the majority of plans made are not implemented, and even those that are, are usually not implemented as originally planned (Harari, 1995; Stacey, 1992). Medical treatment is no different, probably for the same reasons.

In many cases patients do not heed advice or take medication as prescribed, and even when they do, treatment is often not completed. An important reason is that those who have to live the consequences of treatment (patients) often do not understand what they have to do and why. Medicine, like business and technology, operate upon a belief of an organismic metaphor of control. Physicians, as the brain, tell patients what to do and monitor their actions. Patients are not considered to be purposeful individuals or individually responsible once they become part of the health care system. They are supposed to follow instructions, not to understand them. Incomplete treatment is inefficient and a cause of increased cost, and can only be improved by aligned self-control. A prerequisite for this is improved communication between physicians and patients, a different attitude towards illness and health, and a belief in a social system metaphor of control.

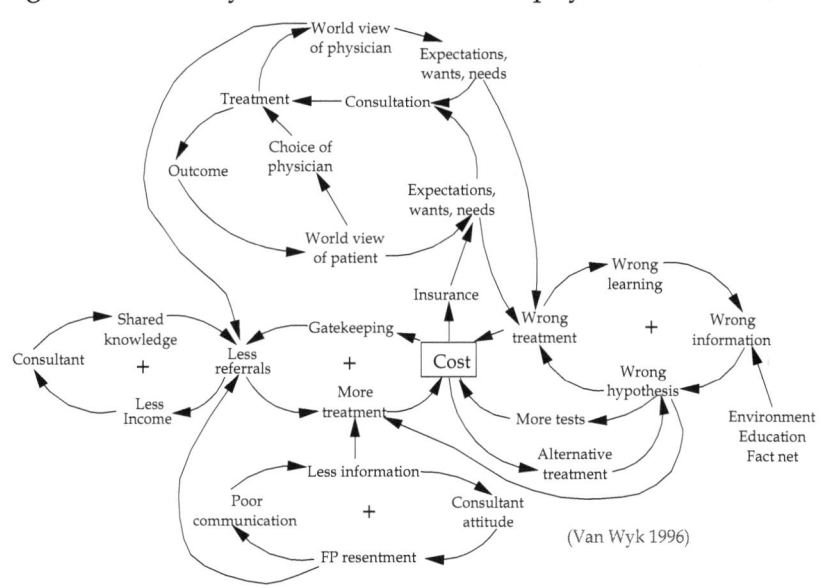

Diagram 24: The Dynamics of the Patient-physician Interaction

(Van Wyk 1996)

Many treatments require the efficient interaction of a number of role players in the health care system, and the process may break down at any point along this chain. When this happens, the result may be tragedy. In terms of process, a highly efficient interaction and a high degree of responsibility (as understood by Vickers) is required by all the components of the system. And again, this can be achieved by the application of systems thinking.

Synthesis

The interactions of the patient-physician system described can be illustrated graphically in a system dynamics model. (See **diagram 24**).

The illustration can be summarized as follows:

- The worldview that physicians have of illness, health care and their own roles, contributes to their expectations, wants and needs. The latter becomes part of the consultation in the ways discussed. The consultation leads to treatment that in turn reinforces the worldview. The worldview is shaped to a large extent by the physician's environment and in the case of family practitioners contributes to referral patterns.
- The outcome of treatment contributes to the worldview of illness and health care that patients have, which in turn is the patient's contribution to the consultation. This worldview also determines the patient's selection of physician, which in turn has an effect on treatment. As discussed, this worldview is shaped mainly under the influence of the patient's environment.
- The expectations, needs and wants of both patients and physicians can lead to incorrect treatment, which has a negative effect on cost. Patient expectations are also influenced by the amount that they have to contribute to health insurance, which in turn is linked to health care cost.
- The amount of correct information and knowledge introduced during the diagnostic cycle has a large influence on the correctness of the hypothesis (diagnosis). A poverty of information is compensated for by more tests, which negatively influence cost. More importantly, incorrect diagnoses lead to incorrect treatment that in turn leads to wrong learning and therefore contribute towards a reinforcing cycle. The quality of information is decided by factors such as the environment, the diagnostic cycle, education and existing fact nets as discussed.
- Gatekeeping is a response to cost that is out of control. It can lead to late referrals and therefore more difficult problems, more treatment and more cost. It therefore contributes toward a reinforcing cycle. Furthermore, gatekeeping reduce the number of referrals that leads to a reduced income for specialists and therefore an incentive to increase the amount of work.
- If specialists share their knowledge and experience with referring physicians, referrals may go down with a reduced income and therefore less incentive to share knowledge. There is an attendant incentive to increase the amount of work as a result of this.
- A superior attitude of consultants results in resentment amongst family practitioners that in turn contributes to poor communication and a deficiency of information. The latter contributes towards more than necessary treatment.

- High health care costs are an incentive for patients to try alternative treatments. This is often based upon incorrect diagnoses, which leads to inappropriate treatment and eventually more treatment. It can therefore have a negative influence on cost.

Conclusion

In terms of the discussion the following can be deduced.

- The purpose of the patient-physician interaction is the resolution of the patient's problem (illness).
- This process is initiated during the consultation. This is a highly complex interaction towards which both patients and physicians contribute through their wants, needs and expectations. Assumptions (beliefs) underlying to the consultation are usually unstated. These include beliefs about illness, professionals and the health care system.
- The diagnostic system is the analytical part of the consultation system. The flow and use of knowledge in this system is not efficient at present. This is a barrier to successful diagnosis, learning and research. This could be improved by altering the process into a circular or learning cycle and also by altering the interchange of information in the physician system.
- The decision to treat is the synthesis of the consultation and diagnostic systems and is therefore influenced by the needs, wants and expectations of patients and physicians. The health care environment also has an influence on the decision to treat. Treatment activates complex chains of health care processes that eventually determine the cost to the system.
- Treatment advice is often not followed, which has cost implications. An important reason is poor communication between patients and physicians and hence a lack of incentive from patients to implement the advice given to them.
- It is the proposition of this book that a system of inquiry ought to be used in the patient-physician interaction that will improve the rigor of the decision-making process. Such a system would have to include assumption testing of underlying belief systems, and a method for evaluating the accuracy of empirical medical knowledge.

In order to change the patient-physician system into a learning system, a methodology is needed that takes a broad view of the problem. Such a methodology is the systems approach.

Chapter 9: A Systems Approach To Health Care Planning

The analysis so far followed Churchman's model of inquiry, namely a problem system was identified, analyzed, clearly described, and its history determined. From these insights, a hypothesis was formed, and it remains to inquire into the implications of the hypothesis. In brief the hypothesis states that:

- The health care system is a complex social system, which in turn is a component of a larger society, or its environment.
- Historically the system developed from its origins as a simple system with a single interaction between patient and physician into a highly complex system with multiple interactions between many actors.
- Our thinking and beliefs about health and health care did not develop in parallel to the system's historical development and consequently in our minds health care process is still thought of as a simple linear causal interaction under the control of individual actors.
- The current worldwide cost problem is the result of a number of individual structural factors that interact with each other in a multiple circular recursive manner in ways that destabilizes health care as a system. Planners who attempt to correct the problem by using traditional analytical methods and focusing on structure to the exclusion of the process dimension will therefore make little headway and more often than not their solutions will lead to new problems.
- The patient-physician interaction is the basic interaction that sets into motion the processes that will eventually determine cost. This interaction is dependent on the needs, wants, and expectations (ends) of both patients and physicians on the one hand, and available knowledge and skills (means) on the other. It is a highly complex interaction that could be improved by an approach that can increase the ability of patients and physicians to understand how their actions affect the system in which they participate. Such knowledge may help to align their mind maps and learning and result in a more efficient system, and at the same time the process of inquiry may contribute towards the improvement of the knowledge, skills, and decision-making ability of physicians.

The rest of this chapter is devoted to exploring the possible effects of applying a systems approach to the health care system. The focus will be on the areas identified as problematic in the patient-physician interaction, namely:

i. The existing worldview, or mind map of health, illness and health care; and
ii. The inefficient use of knowledge in the system.

In keeping with the systems philosophy, proposals in this chapter represent inquiry from the planner's perspective and cannot be prescriptive since in the end a complete inquiry must include the perspectives of clients and decision-makers as well. The purpose of the study is therefore to stimulate thinking about health care planning from within a systems perspective and not to serve as a formula or panacea that will cure health care's problems overnight.

The patient-physician system as a learning system

The objective of group learning as stated before is to test shared images and assumptions (mind maps), and in the case of healthcare the most important assumption to test is that of our worldview of health and health care. The reason for this is that it will make the roles that patients and physicians play in relation to the system more explicit, and they will therefore be able to better recognize the effect of their actions on the system as a whole. The fact that they do affect the system in a negative way was identified as a key cause of the health care cost crisis. The overall objective of inquiry therefore is to achieve aligned self-control of the individual parts of the system and creating a shared vision of how health care ought to be organized, something that becomes possible via the experience gained from a process of inquiry. Such a process by definition results in learning.

An example of a shared vision is the existing worldview of health care, illness and professionals, shared by patients and physicians. The current paradigm was identified as the product of the history of the health care system and is based on a simplistic linear causality model of illness. The question is, what would happen if this worldview could be changed and how would that influence processes in the system?

A systems model of health care

For the purpose of this study it is appropriate to consider a candidate worldview of health and health care from within the framework of a systems approach, which for the purpose of this text will assume that:

- Illness cannot be eradicated from society, but it can be transformed.

- Health can only be defined in terms of the context of a complex system with multiple factor circular causality.
- The treatment of illness takes place within a complex social system.
- Effective planning and intervention in the health care system becomes possible if it is based on a worldview that recognizes the complexity and systemic nature of illness and its treatment.

Diagram 25: The Prevalence of Illness in Society

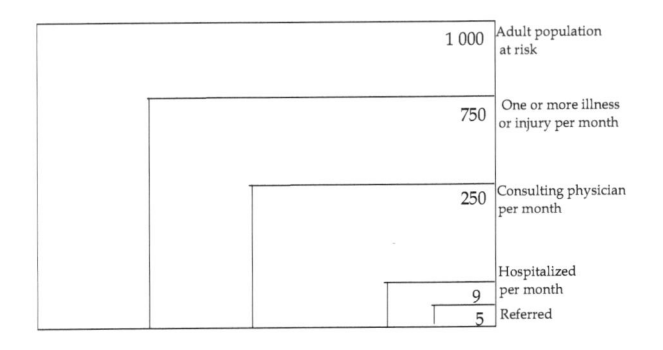

1 000	Adult population at risk
750	One or more illness or injury per month
250	Consulting physician per month
9	Hospitalized per month
5	Referred

White et al. The ecology of medical care. *NEJM (1961)*, 265, 885-892.
Copyright © 1961 Massachusetts Medical Society. All rights reserved.
Reproduced with permission.

White et al (1961) and Green et al (2001) published the results of studies on the prevalence of illness in two different communities in the USA and UK (**diagram 25**). It indicated that out of every 1000 adults in a population, 750 - 800 will experience symptoms of unwellness during a month, but only 210 - 250 will seek medical care, 8 - 9 will be admitted to hospital, and 5 will be referred to another physician. The study implies that the majority of people in a population are likely to experience some symptoms of unwellness such as a sprain, a cold, headache, mild depression, and so on from time to time, but not so that it requires professional care. In other words, it means that the largest number of "ill"[1] people is *inside* the community but outside of the boundaries of the traditional health care system, and that the community is able to deal with them effectively without interference from the medical community. People only become patients and part of the health care treatment system when measures to cope within the framework of the social environment fail.

---

[1] Illness here is considered to be the same as being unwell.

Vickers' model of health care

Vickers (1984) developed a theme along similar lines according to which he distinguishes between:

- Community medicine
- Inpatient medicine; and
- Environmental medicine.

Community medicine has to do with all the resources used for managing illness inside the community, inpatient medicine with the resources devoted to caring for illness in hospitals, and environmental medicine with the resources used for the preventing of illness caused by interacting with the environment. Accordingly, the purpose of inpatient medicine is to return patients to the community where they can continue with self-care as soon as possible, since illness negatively affects other systems in the community such as the family, employment, and so on as well. This suggests that the ability of the community to deal with illness inter alia also depends on its ability to deal with the circumstances that caused the disturbance. By extension therefore, the role of community medicine is to help increase the ability of the community to deal with the circumstances surrounding illness.

Vickers' model implies a drastic rethink of the existing situation, including a different method for selecting candidates for medical school, a different curriculum for training physicians that reflects the principles of the proposed system, and a change in the worldview of physicians and patients.

The implication of both models described above is that the totality of existing health care structures in reality only deals with the needs of approximately 25% of the total community, including the hospital component (about 10%) and the specialist component (about 5%). In other words, the existing illness paradigm focuses exclusively on the group of people within the hospital-consultation (inpatient medicine) system, and ignores the environment of the problem and the structure and purpose of the system as a whole completely. The outcome necessarily is a worldview that assumes hospital-based health care is the only source of good quality care (Rothman, 1997).

A systems model of health

White et al's data can be graphically rearranged in terms of Vickers' model and illustrated on a bell curve (see **diagram 26**). The distribution of patients on this curve and its interpretation is a valid representation of reality and can therefore serve as basis for a more comprehensive, or systems worldview of health care. This model will serve as the dialectic alternative to the existing health care paradigm and as basis to show how using this model could affect the health care system in general in a positive manner.

Diagram 26: A Systems Model of Health

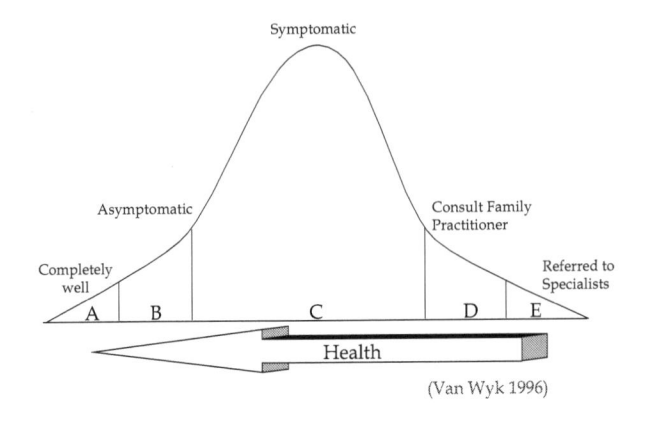

(Van Wyk 1996)

The approach to this concept falls under the rubric of ideals planning, in other words how an ideal health care system could look like. It assumes that illness cannot be removed from society, but that the illness profile can be altered. In terms of this curve, illness, or health in society can be visualized as consisting of a spectrum ranging from the perfectly healthy to the terminally ill. The basis is a continuum rather than traditional either-or healthy-ill binary thinking associated with the Cartesian system, and it is therefore not possible to determine exactly a point at which a person passes from healthy to ill. In fact, exact knowledge of this point is irrelevant. What is of greater importance is how and *why* people move along the continuum from health to illness and back. In other words, what are the reasons why society can no longer deal with the problem itself (by transferring responsibility to the health care treatment system), and how does the health care treatment system cope with the problem in terms of its purpose, or what it ought to do?

For this model, the causes of illness are assumed to be based on a model of complex causality with numerous interactions and feedback between multiple co-producers. This implies that illness as an entity is the product of instability in a highly complex system of interactions and that this should be reflected in treatment. Accordingly, it is more important to see the physician as a *manager* of the complex problem of illness, rather than an expert that can control sequences of simple problems, a concept that will be discussed again later in the text.

The interpretation of the systems model of health is as follows.

- Approximately 25% of a community is healthy without symptoms at a particular moment in time (Groups A and B). Of them about 10% are in perfect health (Group A), and the remainder are asymptomatic but have the potential to become ill (Group B), in other words they wear spectacles, have minor congenital abnormalities, and engage in unhealthy activities such as cigarette smoking, bungee jumping, unsafe sex and so on.
- Group C represents the 50% of a population that suffer from minor symptoms that require no treatment, or that can be dealt with by self-medication.
- The remaining 25% (Groups D and E) constitutes patients under the care of health care professionals, in other words those people that society can no longer cope with without professional help.

The fundamental question in terms of the systems model of health is why did patients progress from A to D/E on the illness continuum, and more importantly, how can they be assisted back into the self care Group (C). The purpose of the patient-physician system in terms of the systems model of health therefore is to assist patients to move along the health continuum from the symptomatically ill group (Groups D and E) to the symptomatically well group (Group C) as speedily and efficiently as possible (Vickers, 1984).

The traditional health care system assumes that family practitioners and specialists are both part of a single system of physicians, but in the systems model of health they are functionally separable in terms of the purpose they ought to fulfill. In terms of this argument, the purpose of specialists is to move referred and hospitalized patients (Group E) as efficiently as possible to the non-hospitalized group (D), that is to the care of family practitioners. Functionally, the outcome is a physician *network* and an altered physician referral system.

The health care system as a purposeful system

In terms of a social system metaphor and the systems model of health, the health care system does not currently accurately reflect the purpose it ought to fulfill in society. Purpose was defined before as the ability to select one's own objectives and the means for pursuing them, and within the confines of this definition, then discussion refers to:

- The purpose of the patient-physician system
- The purpose of its parts (patients, physicians, hospitals, administrators and pharmacists); and

- The purpose of the healthcare system as a whole of which the patient-physician system is a part.

The patient-physician system

The objective of the patient-physician (treatment) system is to maximize the physical and mental capabilities of patients to enable them to function as efficiently as possible. Patients select physicians as the means for achieving this purpose, and physicians in turn use their knowledge and skills, hospital facilities, and pharmaceuticals as their means for assisting patients back towards a state of functional health. An additional means is the financial resources for paying for the services needed to achieve objectives, in the case of economically advantaged patients via medical insurance, and for the less fortunate via the government tax base.

The selection of the correct means, or in other words the right physician, given the confines of the decision environment (ability to pay, availability of physician pool, and so on), is particularly important in order to achieve the best possible outcome.

Physicians

The purpose of physicians, in terms of the systems model of health is to serve as the means for returning patients to a physically and mentally well state so that they can live their lives to their full capacity. However, physician behavior is often determined by their own personal purposes and personal need satisfaction towards achieving individual ends such as financial success, or professional credibility. Traditionally, the unstated assumption is that personal physician ends are subservient to patient needs, however, the social laboratory is not value-free and the values of physicians as treatment planners not only influence but also ought to be considered consciously during decision-making.

Patients

There does not appear to be a clear indication of the health care ends that patients (or society in general) desire, and much of it today is contrived. Evidence exists that patients are interested in knowing more about health issues, but little is done to change the traditionally passive patient role (Greenfield et al., 1985; McNeil et al., 1982). Consequently, patients currently do not and are not expected to participate in decision-making and do not get to understand medical processes or the logic of treatment. That business interests can change the mind maps of people is a well-known fact in the marketing industry. For example Blue Cross in the USA responded to the fiscal crisis affecting hospitals after the Depression with a marketing approach to convince patients that the best treatment is given in hospitals, which is still part of the worldview of health and the cost crisis (Rothman, 1997).

A study conducted amongst patients and physicians supports Arrow's (1963) contention that the health care commodity in actual fact is knowledge (Van Wyk, 2001). In keeping with this argument, patients consult physicians because they want to know the reason for their symptoms and whether the condition they suffer from is serious. Patients mostly expect reassurance and can live with their symptoms if they know their condition is not serious or harmful, and they expect to be advised to take medication or have surgery only if really necessary, or if the condition is serious or potentially harmful[2].

Because patients lack the commodity (knowledge) to begin with, i.e. they have no way of verifying the truth of advice, they expect physicians to make the treatment decision on their behalf and unconditionally trust them to act in their best interest. The fact that only 42% of patients actually follow the advice given to them (Korsch and Negrete, 1973) may be because they did not expect treatment and therefore felt it is unnecessary to take it.[3]

Ends can be divided into needs (that must be fulfilled), and wants (that do not). In terms of Churchman's approach, ends could be goals, objectives, or ideals. The purpose of patient needs is to maximize capabilities, hence to have illness or disability restored to a state where it becomes possible to function socially in an acceptable manner. If needs are not restored, disability, disfigurement, or death may occur. Need satisfaction therefore is usually a goal. However, need satisfaction can also be an objective or ideal when measures are taken to prevent illness from occurring in the future, such as vaccination, efforts to stop smoking, a healthier lifestyle, and so on.

The dilemma is with wants, the attainment of which is not a necessity, and which are shaped largely by expectations, which in turn are shaped by experience and the environment (for example the press). Wants could be a goal, for example the desire to have a small upturned nose, which may be satisfied immediately if the necessary means are available. More problematic is the prevailing worldview of health care, which assumes that in time science will be able to offer society a world free of illness, pain, deformity,

---

[2] Physicians on the other hand believe patients expect treatment, i.e. they think patients think they want treatment although this is not the case, and are therefore likely to be biased towards action rather than inaction. Therefore, when Frankel (1991) and Samuelson (1994) state that unlimited patient wants is an important cost driver, in terms of this study they speak on behalf of physicians rather patients and Illich's (1976), Relman's (1991) and Rothman's (1997) contention that demand is supplier driven instead is more correct.

[3] More often than not, they are right.

disability, ageing, and maybe eventually even death. Wants of this nature obviously contribute to the health care crisis, and not to health.

The deterministic worldview also assumes the ability to fund wants indefinitely in a value-free manner that does not consider the possibility that wants may not be desirable. The satisfaction of wants is an individual pursuit and the attainment limited by a resource, namely funding. The result is a Village Commons problem and to solve the problem competitors in future will have to co-operate i.e. determine communal needs and wants and the resources available for their satisfaction and balance that with individual wants. However, needs and wants often overlap and the problem is who determines whether the purpose is a need or a want? It is in this arena that modern bio-ethics became disorientated as will be discussed later. In sum, there is an underlying tension in health care where the freedom to choose ends conflict with our ability to do so in terms of the description of purpose.

A solution to the problem is to conceive of the health care system as a complex social system. If all participants in the system share a social system worldview of health care, self-alignment becomes possible, which could lead to improved knowledge of the system and therefore a resolution of the needs-wants dilemma.

The physician network system

The role of specialists is compatible with Vickers' inpatient medicine, and his suggestion that the training of this group of physicians ought to concentrate on the traditional illness model (traditional medical training), makes sense in terms of the systems model of health. The fundamental redefinition is towards the role of family practitioners.

In the systems model of health, family practitioners become specialists in their own right (Rakel, 1990) and ought to be trained to fulfill this purpose[4]. Instead of being the barrier (gatekeeper) between specialist, hospital and community, they now have an important role as facilitators. And their purpose becomes to connect to the specialist-hospital system as efficiently as possible and to receive back patients into the community and continue with care commenced in hospital until the patient is symptomatically well. I.e. they become community physicians in Vickers' terms, rather than generalists as at present.

In response to this requirement, the nature of the referral system changes to a network of purposeful physicians (a physician system), rather than the existing linear system and community of separate individual professionals (**diagram 27**). The change is towards professional *teams* with a better chance

---

[4] I.e. they bridge hospital care and the community.

to decide on appropriate treatment protocols and developing more efficient routines (Teisberg and Porter, 1994). Teams will also be able to define protocols appropriate to a particular geographical area and for facilities available to it, rather than having it determined by a distant bureaucracy who do not have to implement it. In this model, purposeful interaction becomes a necessity and could assist in testing communal assumptions and therefore group learning. In other words, this model alters the physician system into a complex social system as well as a learning organization.

Diagram 27: The Physician Network System

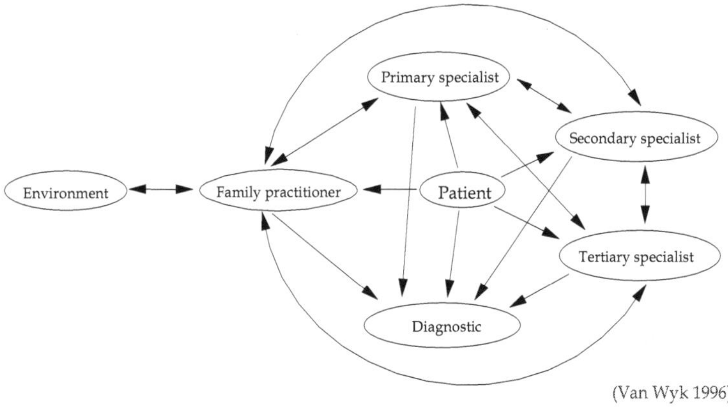

(Van Wyk 1996)

A core requirement for a successful network is the continuous and efficient flow of communication between all its parts (Rakel, 1990), and a network therefore has the potential to break down the existing barriers of communication between physicians, as well as between patients and physicians. The functioning of the network in a way becomes an economies of scale model, because the physical location of family practitioners is less important than contact with the communities they serve and the network. It may be that such an approach could encourage a more equitable distribution of family practitioners in time.

In a network patients do not necessarily have to be referred to specialists, but specialists have an obligation to refer patients to family practitioners for bridging care, and also a duty to ensure that family practitioners have the necessary knowledge and information to continue with care. The network concept recognizes the need for mutual trust and the status of family practitioners as community specialists, which may help to resolve the existing conflict between family practitioners and specialists.

In terms of the systems model of health, community medicine, primary health care, and non-traditional medicine, has a relevant role to play in self-care and the prevention of illness. In other words in this model their purpose is to prevent people from moving from left to right on the continuum by attending to those factors in the environment that can help to prevent people from falling ill (Groups B and C).

The role of non-traditional medicine is to support self-care in patients in Group C. In the traditional health care system these groups are often in conflict with the Western tradition, but in terms of the systems model of health they do have a particular role to play. The model also suggests the role of government, as a major role player in preventative medicine and primary health care, is in ensuring that patients in Groups B and C remain healthy. In other words they are responsibility for implementing measures that will improve the health of society as a whole. This would be represented by Vickers' environmental health.

Information and knowledge

A very important outcome of a physician network is that it also results in an *information* network, which has implications for the distribution of knowledge and implementation of learning systems in health care. In some areas there are no medical schools or medical libraries, consequently physicians exchange a minimal amount of information academically or otherwise. And yet, there are often numerous specialists, each with a large amount of learning, experience, and personal libraries filled with textbooks and the latest journals. The question is how can this knowledge be accessed, and the answer is by the breaking down of barriers to communication.

The redefined purpose of specialists in a network includes a vital role in the dissemination of information, and knowledge. They can be consulted not only towards the resolution of illness, but also as disseminators of knowledge. Furthermore, an important role of the specialist (in Vickers' terms) is to research more effective treatments (traditional research) and also to determine how well preventative measures worked to prevent illness from progressing towards the hospital system (Donaldson, 1992).

Rutstein et al (1976) described an interesting method to measure exactly this sort of outcome based on the principle that:

- Quality is the effect of care on the health of the individual and the population as a whole and is therefore concerned with outcomes.

- Efficiency is an index of how well the health care system functions and is therefore concerned with process.

For the purpose of this method, illnesses are grouped into three classes based on norms agreed on by "experts" in the field.

- Group 1 represents those illnesses that ought to be investigated as indicators of quality and health when a single case occurs. The illness that occurred caused disability or death, because it was not prevented or treated properly.
- Group 2 concerns illnesses that lead to investigation when more than one case occurs, in other words there is a pattern of illness as a result of inadequate prevention or treatment.
- Group 3 includes illnesses of which the effect on quality and efficiency is not yet known and therefore need further study.

A single case of illness from Group 1 or number of cases of illnesses listed in Group 2 may indicate inefficiency (preventative measures failed), or poor quality (poor treatment was given). Not enough is known about illnesses in Group 3 at this stage, and more data is necessary before their significance can be determined. It would appear as if this approach is appropriate to a systems model of health and more relevant for monitoring the efficiency of health care than existing medical audits.

In principle, outcomes measurements are measures of performance, hence, they indicate whether patient ends were successfully achieved, and in terms of this argument Rutstein's method is an excellent measure of the success with which the system achieved patients' purpose. It determines for a systems model of health whether the system successfully prevented patients from moving towards symptomatic illness, and whether it successfully returned patients to the asymptomatic group. It is less successful as a measure of wants fulfillment, since this is largely determined by patient satisfaction.

The problem with traditional measures of performance such as audit is that they are concerned only with treatment outcomes, and designed on an assumption of simple linear causal interactions. Therefore they may apply as measures of performance of process, but they fail as measures of the performance of whole systems.

Networks in practice

Physician networks may be constructed in a number of ways towards which the following principles may contribute.

Large health care organizations have the resources and are positioned in such a way that they are able to contract only physicians committed to the principles of a shared vision (Kronick et al. 1993). At present, managed care organizations identify physician practices for contracting that show efficient utilization of resources, which has shortcomings as regards implementation (Milstein et al. 1989). Also, the role of managed care organizations in contracting selected physicians is a contentious issue since it may lead to rationing and the loss of some high-technology treatments. However, it could also ensure that only self-aligned individuals with a commitment to learning will be part of the organization with the opportunity to implement planning and to proceed according to the objectives identified as desirable earlier. A commitment to exchange knowledge and learning is a fundamental principle without which the proposed model will be difficult to implement.

Closer co-operation between physicians is likely to lead to better practice (Rakel, 1990). Specialists in particular have a responsibility to share their knowledge with family practitioners and other colleagues through personal contact. This in turn may lead to improved interpersonal communication and familiarity, hence, such exchanges may break down the existing barrier of anonymity (Balint, 1986). It could also serve as basis for mutual respect and an understanding of the role, purpose, and effects of decision-making of each individual actor on the system as a whole (Milstein et al. 1989), i.e. it could satisfy the systems condition of participation. The ideal is achievable through clinical discussion groups and a requirement that physicians who participate in the system should obtain a minimum number of attendance credits in order to ensure their continued participation in the system.

Traditionally, medical practice is executed in great secrecy. This attitude is shaped to a large extent by the legal requirement of patient confidentiality and reinforced by the regulations of medical councils (who interpret the value system of the profession). The result is suspicion and a lack of communication. Studies indicated that showing physicians how their practices compare to the average patterns for a geographic area or specialty free of value judgments is more effective in changing practice patterns than general methods of education (Milstein et al. 1989). The implication is that transparency and breaking down the traditional barriers to communication help physicians to form an understanding of how the way they practice influence the system.

In summary, in the preceding section the prevailing worldview of health care was challenged by an alternative, namely the systems model of health. The latter is based on a profile of illness as it actually occurs in society and may therefore better reflect reality. The application of this worldview affects health care in the following ways:

i. Shared beliefs about health and health care are changed into a more systemic comprehensive image and a better reflection of reality.
ii. The model converts the health care system into the complex social system that it is based on a shared vision and understanding.
iii. The role of physicians is redefined as a community of physicians of which the purpose is to manage illness as a complex biological and social problem.
iv. In a physician network knowledge can be utilized more efficiently.
v. This model of health is more conductive to learning than the existing system.

The health care system in terms of Churchman's methodology

Clients (the source of motivation)

In the traditional treatment system, the following clients can be identified who benefit directly from the interaction (Teisberg and Porter, 1994).

1. *Patients*, whose purpose is to get the best quality of health care regardless of cost, and whose measure of performance is a satisfactory outcome of treatment. When a need is fulfilled, the illness will have been cured or contained, but the measure in terms of wants is the satisfaction of expectations. Due to the difficulties inherent in the sharing of mind maps, the satisfaction of expectations is sometimes difficult to ascertain and dissatisfaction, because of a mismatch of ideas, can easily lead to disillusionment and legal difficulties. This is in contrast to need satisfaction where legal difficulties will be as a result of omission or negligence.
2. *Physicians*, whose purpose is to provide treatment to patients, i.e. make their knowledge and skills available, and to earn the maximum possible income in return. Their measure of performance is professional status and income, although there still are some physicians who feel called in the historical sense to serve their communities and whose measure of performance is personal satisfaction.
3. *Administrators*, whose purpose is to spend less on health care than they receive in premiums or taxes, and their measure of performance is a balanced budget and a sufficient profit to ensure the continued existence of the organization. In modern private health care systems administrators are often employees of for-profit organizations, whose measure of performance is profit for distribution to shareholders. This creates a value dilemma, is it acceptable for excess funds, or funds generated by savings in the health care system to be distributed to people who are not beneficiaries of the system? In a free market model, the argument is that such funds are reinvested in new health care ventures,

but there does not appear to be convincing proof for this. Furthermore, who determines that optimum reinvestment will occur in a socially responsible way?
4. *Health care systems* (hospitals and pharmacists), whose purpose it is to make facilities available to physicians for treating patients and whose measure of performance is profit. In the case of government institutions the aim is not profit, but at the present time cost containment and a balanced budget.
5. Other clients are parts of the larger health care system and the social system in general. For example patient employers who contribute towards health care insurance and whose purpose is to pay the lowest premium to medical administrators that will retain satisfied employees. These clients are not within the boundaries selected for this study.

The client in a systems model of health

Who would the clients be when the worldview of health care is altered to a systems model of health and what ought their purpose and measure of performance to be?

1. The purpose of *patients* in a systems model of health is to remain in the asymptomatic or symptomatically well group of the community (Groups A, B or C), and the measure of performance is their ability to fulfill this purpose within the community as efficiently as possible. This may result in a community that benefits from the ability of its members to live their lives to their full capabilities, in other words satisfy Blum's definition of health care referred to earlier. Such a state of affairs could lead to the betterment of society as a whole, where everyone benefits from the fitness of its members.
2. The purpose of *physicians* in terms of this model is to move patients from the hospitalized and symptomatic groups (Groups D and E) back into the community. The measure of performance ought to be a minimum number of patients at any one time in the treatment system, in other words the opposite of the present system. The problem with such a change in worldview is the fear of a loss of income. But it is possible to allay this fear with a remuneration system that rewards the purpose of physicians in alignment with a systems model of health (rather than for time as at present), as will be shown.

Neither patients nor physicians have the resources to implement planning, which is why they qualify as clients and planners who ought to benefit from the system, but not decision makers in a systems sense. In terms of Ulrich's modification of Churchman's methodology, patients and physicians are affected by decision-making and therefore ought to be the beneficiaries of planning. They may be enabled to learn about the results of their actions on the system, and also be ensured that their ideals and values are incorporated in design (the source of motivation) by involving them in planning. Participative planning may therefore lead to a more efficient system (lower cost) and better implementation.

In the traditional health care model there is a needs-wants dilemma described earlier, which needs to be resolved at the level of the patient as client, in other words at community level, since it involves the purpose of the community. Integration of the purposes of the community and patients in terms of a social system model has a direct effect on the patient-physician interaction, and could resolve the present tension between personal wants and communal needs. The problem is that when there are limited resources, not everyone can share in it, and the question then becomes, should it be denied to everyone including those who can afford it? (Donaldson, 1992) I.e. there is a tension between what is good for the patient and what is good for society (Fuchs, 1984). Inequality is a consequence of the distribution of social advantage and inequality in health care is a reflection of this reality. Hence, the redistribution of resources denies people with a social advantage the ability to buy health wants, given the fact that the amount of "health" that social advantage can buy is a matter of debate. (Indications are that education, skills, and an expanding economy is more important for achieving health than intervention by the health care treatment system).

A different way to approach the problem is to ask who is the source of expertise that can resolve the needs-wants dilemma? In terms of the argument so far, needs are about illness and the experts about illness by definition is physicians, therefore physicians may plan patient needs. On the other hand, wants are a value issue and there are no experts on values, hence the source of expertise in this case is patients themselves. Individual wants lead to the exhaustion of limited funding, the common resource, therefore, the solution to the wants dilemma is the resolution of the individual versus communal wants tension referred to earlier in the text. And the application of the systems model of health may facilitate this.

A situation where all the members of a community have unrestricted access to all possible treatments is an ideal (De Wet, 1991)[5] that cannot be achieved, but in terms of ideals planning it can be approached indefinitely. To begin with therefore, planning must address what can be achieved with available resources in a moral and ethical way.

---

[5]This is the often-quoted ideal of an equitable distribution of health care. The achievement of this is an ideal that cannot be attained within present socio-economic realities (De Wet, 1991).

Planners (the source of expertise)

The following entities and institutions presently participate and dominate health care planning.

1. *Governments* as planners traditionally contribute no expertise towards planning and therefore assemble boards of inquiry whose purpose is to provide them with plans to solve their problems. The dilemma is to select the right panel and to guarantee that these members in fact have the necessary expertise. Selection often shows political bias in order to satisfy predetermined policy positions, i.e. plans are often formulated to satisfy the aims of ruling parties. The aim is short-term, or goals planning, and the ultimate purpose is to secure re-election. Government planning is often constrained by specified time limits, lack of funding, specified parameters that limit the scope of inquiry, and difficulties in assimilating the views of all those involved by the possible outcomes of planning. In other words, the approach suffers from the usual shortcomings of goals planning, of which the most serious is a lack of attention to values and ethics and the specified limitations that inhibit the scope of inquiry. Goals planning cannot guarantee that society will benefit from the plans, since the underlying metaphor is mechanismic.
2. *Business'* approach to health care planning is whatever is necessary to control and secure a profit, i.e. the application of business "science". It is based on the assumption that health care cannot manage itself and business can offer the necessary expertise to do this for them. It also assumes that management principles that apply to business can apply to health care. Planning therefore consists of finding ways to adapt these principles for use in the health care system. The approach again is goals planning and therefore, again, there is no guarantee that business science will be of benefit to the health care system and society in general. The operative metaphor is organismic.
3. *Social scientists* plan for health care in academic and other institutions. They have an important contribution to make to the process of inquiry, however, their paradigm for now is the scientific metaphor, which restricts their ability to address the complexity of the health care system.
4. *Medical associations* representing physicians, their aspirations, and values potentially have an important role to play in planning, which unfortunately does not happen. They have the power to alter the worldview of their membership and therefore potentially the whole health care system, but the purpose of their planning currently is to protect the status quo.
5. *Systems planners* require all of the stakeholders to participate in planning the system, including patients, physicians, administrators, government, and so on. Participation in planning and inquiry may lead to aligned self-control and a changed worldview. The method is ideals planning and

ought to include the aspirations and values of all stakeholders, in other words the aim is to align purposes. Since planning is never complete, the process is a never-ending cycle of planning and learning. Furthermore, in a rapidly changing environment plans are often obsolete by the time that they are implemented and therefore have to be continuously adjusted. A shared vision of health care is the best guarantee that the members of the system will agree to implement potentially beneficial changes. The planner in this model is whoever can assist the members of the system to plan for themselves.

The biggest problem of planning is that of implementation. This text proposes that the notion that patients may respond well to participation is feasible, particularly if the idea can be introduced on a smaller scale, in other words at the patient-physician interface. For example, participation may be ensured at the level of consumer groups and the teaching of self-care.

Participation

1. Patients

    The idea that the community ought to partake in health care planning has been championed before by planners of primary health care systems (Shisana and Versfeld, 1993). The problem with the approach is the implicitly stated position that the community should participate in the *management* of their own care, rather than in planning and the result is that community participation has not yet been shown to be of benefit. According to these authors there are potentially three levels of community participation, namely:

    i. Contributing towards predetermined plans (the implementation of goals planning).
    ii. Representation in organizational structures (power sharing).
    iii. Community empowerment to make decisions about their own affairs (self-reliance), which in principle approximates a systems approach, although the context is management rather than planning.

    Community participation is meant to occur at the primary care level, in other words Groups A to C of the systems model of health. However, community participation as conceived of here is without the benefit of a clear worldview of illness, health, and health care systems. Shisana and Versfeld's model also suggests that representatives for the community can be substituted by elected politicians who can then plan on their behalf. This is an erroneous belief since politicians are elected on the basis of a political system of which the predominant metaphor is power, and not sharing.

In a systems model of health it *does* become possible for patients to participate in planning if family practitioners are made responsible for involving their patients in a learning system in terms of the framework of responsibility proposed by the model. They are in a position to teach patients skills of self-medication, preventative medicine, and so on during the patient-physician interaction. Knowledge can also be transferred to the community through groups of patients that are regularly informed about the effect of their actions, both communally and individually on the community's health care (Nienaber, 1995). In this example, the approach led to significant savings and learning. Another study indicated that educational material included with patient accounts about the proper role of self-care can reduce ambulatory care by 17% (Milstein et al. 1989)[6]. Consumer groups could also become a vessel for effective feedback from the community to planners of the health care system and in this way indirectly solve the problem of community participation in the planning process. At the same time that knowledge is transferred, the community may learn how their actions contribute to the problems in the health care system. Knowledge transfer can therefore contribute towards a learning system for all members of the patient-physician interaction.

2. Physicians

It is important to ensure the participation of physicians, who "control" much of the patient-physician interaction[7]. Two areas will need to be addressed to ensure their co-operation.

i. Agreement on treatment protocols.
ii. Remuneration.

The effect of feedback about practice profiles in controlling physician behavior was shown earlier. Local activities, as suggested by the network model, have the advantage of placing control of the change of process in the hands of the affected physicians and removing the perception that guidelines are outside directives (Lomas et al. 1991). Personalisation is therefore an essential component for effectiveness and is an acceptable systemic position.

The problem of remuneration will be discussed in a next section.

In summary, the notion that participation is desirable is based on a large-scale vision of health care delivery that in turn is based on a comprehensive

---

[6]In traditional communities, the older members of the community taught self-care to the young. The view that physicians should take over this role (which drives up cost) may be the result of a loss of traditional systems in the community.
[7]Decisions made by physicians generate 70 to 80% of health care costs (De Wet, 1991).

or systems approach to health care. The challenge is to secure buy in from physicians and patients to this vision. The vision is not about wholesale changing the health care system, but about seeing it in a different way. The model avoids the problems associated with direct control of physicians and patients. The basis is ideals planning and the time to effect therefore as to be expected is long. However the long-term gain from altering behavior may be better than short-term discomfort.

The decision maker (the source of control)

Decision makers have the means or resources that may enable the implementation of a systems model of health. In the traditional system the following decision makers can be identified:

1. *Governments* control health care resources (physicians, education, pharmaceutical industry, hospitals, and so on) by regulation. The political system has the power to make laws pertaining to the health care system and has the resources (civil service, legal system, tax system, and so on) with which to implement them. In terms of the health care system, they therefore have the means to change its future. However, they are not in control of the complex interactions of social interaction, illness, the patient-physician interaction, and so on, i.e. the total system environment.
2. *Business* controls the important resources that enable treatment (manufacturing of health care products including pharmaceuticals, hospitals, nursing staff, medical insurance, and so on). These resources are used as means for controlling physicians and patients, for example by manipulating funds, and controlling inputs and outputs. Co-producers in the environment beyond their control are the same as for governments.
3. The *medical community* controls the knowledge and skills-base that makes the prevention and treatment of illnesses possible. Additional factors in the environment beyond their control are government and business.
4. In terms of the ideal health care dispensation, patients ought to be decision makers as well. They control many of the co-producers of illness (smoking, bungee jumping, industrial accidents, and so on), and are therefore able to select their own objectives and means for pursuing an improvement in their health. The physicians they select influence not only on the satisfaction of their objectives, but also the cost problem. Their worldview of health and health care therefore ought to be changed to include themselves as decision takers as regards those aspects of illness that they are able to change.

Patients and physicians currently find themselves unable to personally contribute towards correcting the ills of the health care system, although according to the hypothesis of a malfunctioning patient-physician interaction they significantly contribute towards the failure of the system. The reason planners ignore them as decision makers is that they are perceived not to control resources that may help to change the existing paradigm. The question is who else controls these resources and can therefore implement health planning? The two most powerful actors are government and the business community (administrators) and if the aim of planning is to make changes at the patient-physician system level, the latter could have an important role to play.

Government

The mixed-model social insurance type of system described earlier appears to have withstood the problems of health care systems the best, which implies that some sort of regulation to control the system may be beneficial. In a sense, this system represents a dialectical synthesis between the opposites of a free-market system and national health.

The problem of course is to ensure that government policies do not contradict health care policies. For example the USA government subsidizes the tobacco industry and yet, this industry plays a large role in increasing health care costs by causing ill health. Governments therefore must take a broader view in their decision-making to avoid this sort of problem (Teisberg and Porter, 1994).

Governments have the power to change barriers of entry into the medical profession and physician education. They are therefore in a position not only to implement a systems model of health, but also to strongly influence the communal worldview of illness and health, provided they are clear about the model to implement.

Business

The best placed organized structure for changing the patient-physician system into a social systems model is the business community, since It commands a wide range of resources (funds, manpower, infrastructure, and so on) that may be used to change the system into a learning system. Their purpose would be to assist in a venture that could have a profound influence on the health care system in general, and with the potential for large cost savings, i.e. they would ultimately benefit from the interaction. Furthermore, intervention does not require a large investment of money, but rather an investment in time and a belief in the type of vision described in this chapter.

The aim of intervention would be a system that functions more efficiently, in other words more purposefully.

Efficiency

To be efficient[8], the patient-physician interaction must:

- Use resources more efficiently, i.e.
  a) Have communication of a high order; and
  b) Use experience and knowledge in the system effectively.
- Work within a revised model for comprehensive health care, such as the proposed systems model.

A systems model of health and physician network could satisfy these criteria, since a re-structuring of resources could ensure a better functioning whole at a lower cost and with higher quality outcomes (Rutstein et al. 1976). The ways such a system could improve communication between physicians and increase the use of available knowledge was described earlier.

In a network, control of the physician system is no longer the function of a gatekeeper, but as a result of aligned self-control is the responsibility of the network itself. For example, at present radiologists perform many expensive diagnostic procedures that they believe are unnecessary for proper diagnoses. However, if they refuse to do so they will be punished by the remuneration system. If the structure of the system is altered to avoid this problem, the diagnostic disciplines can become gatekeepers in their own right. Similarly, in teaching hospitals the highest hurdle to clear to book a case for surgery is the anesthetic department. Again, in the current system aneasthesiologists cannot afford to fulfill this function. However, in a network system, this discipline could act as a gatekeeper for unnecessary surgery. Which raises another cornerstone of a physician network system, namely remuneration.

Remuneration

Existing private care remuneration systems reward time (Coopers, du Toit, 1991; Coopers, du Toit, 1992) and not the knowledge and skills that physicians use. In other words it does not reward those actions used to fulfill the purpose of physicians. Fee-for-service rewards lead to perverse incentives and abuse and therefore must be changed. The social model of health care in Germany salaries specialists accredited to give hospital treatment and capitates consulting specialists and family practitioners. This is not dissimilar to the British NHS system in which specialists are well salaried and family practitioners capitated as well, but via the government tax base. It is difficult to determine an optimal remuneration method from within the existing rewards paradigm, and a system with multiple options may be the most efficient one.

---

[8] *Efficient*: a) productive with minimum waste or effort; b) capable (Allen, 1992)

An alternative is to specifically reward the efficient use of knowledge and skills. In such a system remuneration would be for diagnosis (knowledge) and procedures (skill) only. The diagnostic fee would be for correctly diagnosing, including additional tools that the physician may decide to use to diagnose such as endoscopy, EEG, urine tests, lung function tests, and so on. At present there is additional reward for using these tests, which in many cases leads to abuse. The proposed system could therefore lead to a large reduction in the use of unnecessary tests, which often is hospital based, and this could result in a large reduction in costs, but not at the expense of physician remuneration. This model does not affect autonomy in decision-making either since the aim is accurate decision-making.

Procedures (skills) may be rewarded according to three scales to reflect the degree of difficulty of skills required, for example minor, intermediate, and high or complicated. The fee would be for successful treatment and therefore includes visits relating to the treatment. It also means that physicians would have to accept the risk for complications and its treatment, for which there would be no additional reimbursement. The risk for unnecessary procedures may be monitored through mandatory second opinions for elective procedures, which in effect is a form of indirect peer review, although this is a controversial issue. The proposed skills reward ought to be a strong motivator for more efficient practice.

The emphasis in a system that rewards knowledge and skills is on quality and efficiency, in other words the system creates an incentive for physicians to use their knowledge and skills more efficiently for the purpose of returning patients to self-care. Such a system is appropriate to a systems model of health.

Finally, the two structures with significant control over financial resources and can therefore alter the remuneration system are governments and business. They are in the position to redesign and implement the remuneration system as part of a comprehensive redesign of the health care system in a way that may contribute towards a more efficient system.

Systems philosophy (the source of legitimation)

The final question according to Churchman is whether the systems approach was successful in planning for improvement. This must include the views of the enemies (politics, religion, aesthetics, and morality) and also show the significance of the plan. Ulrich interprets this to mean the fact that someone should act as witness for the affected who are not part of planning, but who will live the consequences of the it. Therefore the question of meaning and witnessing must be addressed, and it is in this area that the organized medical community could have a large and as yet unaddressed role to play.

The different medical associations have neither statutory rights nor are they functional labor unions. They consequently have neither power over their members, nor real power to negotiate with other parties in the traditional sense. It is the thesis of this text that the role of these organizations ought to be redefined, since at present their role is unclear and mostly appear to be related to tariff negotiations and education. They consequently tend to react to changes in the environment rather than anticipate and influence them.

However, they are in the unique position in that they could potentially play a leading role in redefining the worldview of illness and health (Levinsky, 1984b) particularly amongst its members. In this way they have the opportunity to serve as the conscience of their community. But more importantly, they may play the vital role of being the ethical conscience of the profession by virtue of a shared worldview of illness and health care, whilst acting as the conscience or witness for patients at the same time. In other words they could act as the conscience for the people affected by planning, which also satisfies the dilemma of serving the common good of both the patient and the community (De Wet, 1991). In terms of Churchman's concept of ethics both the community and physicians will benefit from the interaction, thereby enabling both to live out their individual wishes. Such a state of harmony and stability approaches that of the original primitive health care system.

Medical ethics can be defined as inquiry during which the concepts, assumptions, beliefs, attitudes, reasons, and arguments underlying medical-moral decision-making are examined critically (Gillon, 1985). Accordingly, medico-moral decisions concern the values according to which the decision is made whether something is right or wrong, and ought or ought not be done. As of yet, the ideal of a comprehensive moral theory for medical practice based on universal principles applying to all and capable of justifying conduct in individual cases has not been attained. However, from a pragmatic point of view this ideal can be approached infinitely, and it is in this that medical societies have a potential role as moral standard-bearer.

One of the core issues in medical ethics is the way that physicians balance personal against with patient interests (Pellegrino, 1987). For example, do physicians have a duty to treat under all circumstances, and if not, when should they (Gillon, 1985; Pellegrino, 1987), since this could be construed as an intrusion in physician needs and wants. Nowadays, there is a belief that medical practice (and the selling of knowledge and skills) is a business like any other business and business ethics should therefore apply to it, which is untenable for three reasons:

i. Ill people are in a position of weakness and vulnerability, for example they must expose and allow themselves to be touched by strangers in order to be examined, and can therefore be exploited. They have no choice but to trust physicians during their predicament, something that physicians invite when they put their knowledge and skills to the disposal of the ill.
ii. The knowledge that physicians acquire through their education is through the sanction of society.
iii. This creates a moral responsibility towards society, which is acknowledged by the Oath at graduation (Pellegrino, 1987). Thus professing to be a professional is an ethical act (Kass, 1983), during which the physician undertakes not to take advantage of the patient's position of vulnerability.

This ethical position is under continuous attack from the legal profession, government, consumer groups, and others (Kass, 1983; De Wet, 1991). The problem is that these groups themselves contribute to the ethical position (value system) of society as a whole. Ethical decisions are therefore no longer an individual choice, but in many cases becomes a consensual decision between a number of interested parties. Again, the medical profession as the interface between symptomatic illness and society may have a role as the facilitator in this process. The role becomes critical in providing an ethical foundation for health care policy decision-making, since they act as the conscience for the value implications of decision-making.

Finally, the position of the enemies must be considered. It was possible to include the views and concerns of government, business, the social sciences, and so on as part of inquiry into comprehensive plan or solution to the health care dilemma in the proposed systems model of health. The plan is a dialectic synthesis of the positions of the enemies on the one hand and systems philosophy on the other.

Government and managed care regulation in effect are systems for rationing health care (Samuelson, 1993), and in Britain's NHS system rationing is already explicit (Schwartz and Aaron, 1984) by limiting resources, which in turn leads to waiting lists. (The environmental response has been growth of the private sector to accommodate cases that can afford to pay and do not wish to wait). The problem is, who decides which patients get what treatment and who tells them? In the NHS system this responsibility is delegated to physicians, which creates tension between the ethical position of physicians and the reality within which they have to live. Physicians then do not tell patients if a certain treatment is available, which can be the source of friction if the patient discovers the deceit. In Britain, this tension is balanced by the difficulty of litigation, which is the result of the British legal system.

In terms of an ideal of comprehensive health care, rationing in some way for the moment is a reality, but in the long-term may fall away. The reason that rationing and control are instituted is the failure to confront business and government with a better more comprehensive plan. The systems community so far failed to present a convincing alternative. The suggested framework could form the basis for such an alternative, but the co-operation of business and government will be vital for implementation, in other words to assist in changing the minds of the community.

A Churchmanian approach to the diagnosis-treatment system

Churchman's philosophy and methodology has another important potential application, namely in the diagnostic system. If the purpose of the physician is to secure an improvement of the patient's condition, then the physician could be seen as a manager of illness. According to Churchman (1968b), a manager is someone who decides among alternative choices. Physicians prepare a differential diagnosis (alternative diagnoses) before selecting the most promising alternative to implement. They also choose between alternative treatments for the condition that they diagnosed. Whether physicians currently are good managers is a matter of opinion, since finding suitable criteria for identifying best managers is problematic[9]. The critical point is more efficiency during the decision-making process.

If Churchman's method is applied to the patient-physician interaction (refer to **diagram 19**, page 166), the following discussion has relevance.

The environment from which patients and physicians get together to interact may be altered by use a systems model of health. Patients benefit from the interaction through improved health, whereas physicians benefit from growing experience (learning), as well as remuneration for their services. Both are therefore clients of the system.

During the diagnostic cycle the questions, what do I know, and how do I know that what I know is true must be asked repeatedly. The problem is that physicians have to rely on the patient's word that its description of the problem is correct. This subjectivity is tested during the rest of the diagnostic cycle, for example during the physical examination additional information is collected to verify the history. In a way then, the patient-physician interaction can be seen as a social laboratory in which the patient is observed.

The problem is, how objective are physicians when they make their observations, and how can they be certain that what they observe is correct? Furthermore, these observations lead to conclusions based on inductive

---

[9]See *The myth of management* (Churchman, 1968) for a discussion of this problem.

reasoning and if the observation is incorrect, so are the conclusions. Therefore, to gain a better understanding of the information collected during history taking and the physical examination, the additional knowledge the physician has from learning and experience is swept into the inquiry, which is mostly the result of academic learning. The problem then becomes how much knowledge about the condition under study does a physician have, and how was this knowledge acquired and validated?

The answer to this dilemma may be found by using Churchman's inquiring system. Medical knowledge is constructed and combined in fact nets, of which the contingent truths are usually determined empirically and validated by a community of experts. The problems of fact nets and the community of experts were discussed before, and in addition, it is important for physicians to ask what assumptions are that they make about these facts and furthermore to consider alternatives viewpoints. In other words, what alternatives are there to the most likely diagnosis (hypothesis), and what alternative viewpoints are there about the appropriate treatment? A pragmatic approach requires that a diagnosis (decision) is made, but the physician must realize that the decision is based on incomplete knowledge. Therefore, the outcome when the hypothesis is tested (by treatment) must be observed and the hypothesis adjusted until the goal of a cure or improvement is attained. In this way, continuous learning by experience may take place. Furthermore, to approach the ideal of complete knowledge about the condition, a program of continuous post-graduate education is a necessity in order to improve decision-making ability. Churchman's approach confirms the earlier proposal that diagnosis ought to be a cycle of inquiry, rather than the current linear cookbook approach.

If findings cannot be explained, in other words a final diagnosis cannot be made, more information must be swept in. Information may be acquired by additional study, consultation with a colleague, or special investigations. Inquiry can also be broadened to include information about the environment of patients, in other words how their family situation, work situation, and so on contributed to the problem. Family practitioners have a particularly important role to play in this regard in terms of a systems model of health. Data shows that of a normal 15-minute family practitioner consultation, only 6 minutes is spent on inquiry and problem solving (Pistorius and Pistorius, 1986), which in terms of the Churchmanian model is clearly inadequate.

Proof for a diagnosis may be obtained from special investigations. In a rigorous system of inquiry, testing is more purposeful and therefore more efficient in the pragmatic sense, since testing is a measurement proving a hypothesis, rather than a random search for a solution. The difficulties of testing and measurement discussed before must however be kept in mind. For example it is important to remember that medical tests are based only on the statistical probability that a certain measure will be normal if a reading is found to be within a certain range. Not only must the possible degree of error be considered during interpretation, but it is also important to ask the right question to arrive at the correct answer.

The decision to treat has two components, namely a dialectic and a value question. The dialectic is in terms of the appropriateness of treatment. What alternatives are available, and which one or combination is most appropriate to the particular case? What guarantee is there that whatever option is selected will improve the patient's condition (ensure betterment)?

The value question refers to what is in the patient's best interest given his or her particular circumstances. Since patients must live with the consequences of the treatment decision, be it good or bad, they are the experts on value questions and their wishes must therefore be solicited and included in the final treatment decision. Not only must they be fully informed by the physician (expert) about possible outcomes, but physicians must also question their own motives in making a particular decision.

Lastly, the enemy of the treatment must be considered. Is it possible that the patient's expectation, however irrational it may be is a viable solution to the problem? Are the rules imposed by government or managed care in terms of payment or treatment protocol right for this case? Is the decision right in terms of the needs of the larger community?

Reflection on the outcome of treatment is vital for inquiry as a cycle of learning. During reflection more perspectives can be swept in that in turn may result in better understanding and learning.

Ultimately then, the quality of the outcome of treatment is determined by the quality of the decision, since it determines what actions is taken (knowledge), and the quality with which those actions are executed (skill).

According to Eddy (1990a), the goal of the treatment decision ought to be to select the outcome most likely to deliver the outcome that the patient finds desirable[10], in other words to satisfy the measure of performance of the client. To make such a decision two steps are needed, namely estimating the:

i. Outcomes of alternative options (is the treatment feasible?); and
ii. Desirability of alternative options (is the treatment desirable?), i.e.
    a) The benefit of options compared to the potential harm (risks, side-effects, inconvenience, and so on) to the patient.

---

[10]Eddy's work is based upon the traditional health care and illness models. Here however, the model is used in terms of the systems model of health.

b) Outcomes compared to the cost of each options (an the health care system afford the treatment?); and
c) If resources are limited, options likely to have the highest yield in terms of outcome must be prioritized (affordability).

Ultimately, the treatment decision is therefore a question of balancing values and preferences. Patients have to live (or die) with outcomes and therefore are the sole experts of what the appropriate treatment is for them. Fact is that due to the complexity and incompleteness of knowledge, in medicine there is no single right or wrong answer. The role of physicians as planners, or experts, is therefore to supply patients (clients) with the best possible information to arrive at a decision. Physicians contribute the empirical component, but patients add the value component to the treatment decision. In an ideals based system, decision-making therefore ought to be the product of the *interaction* between patient and physician. In effect, physicians attempt to present possible scenarios of outcomes based on their inquiry into the illness, which may assist patients to select the most appropriate option for them.

Errors occur in decision-making occur if there is a misperception of the possible outcome, or of the patient's values (**table 7**) (Eddy, 1990a).

Table 7: Error in decision-making

Misperceptions of outcomes occur when:	Misperceptions of preferences occur when:
• Important outcomes are ignored • Extraneous outcomes are included • Available evidence of an outcome is incomplete • Existing evidence is overlooked • Evidence is misinterpreted • Personal experience is too heavily weighted • Wishful thinking	• Patients misunderstand an outcome • The measure of the outcome is misleading • The outcome is presented in ways that lead to different conclusions • The patient is not consulted at all (the usual situation) • Physicians project their own preferences on the patient

The participation of the patient in decision-making is important, for if patients elect to delegate the decision to the planner and decision maker (physician), the latter assumes responsibility for projecting not their own, but the patient's values onto the process. This is only possible within a model with a strong ethical base and a desire to improve the patient's condition in a responsible way, and Churchman's approach can make a significant contribution in this regard.

Summary

- Both patients and physicians are clients of the diagnostic system, and the operative model of health care determines their purpose and measure of performance.
- Physicians are expert planners contracted to achieve the goal of a healthy patient. The reason patients do not complete prescribed courses of medication, or take their prescriptions as prescribed is partially because patients do not understand illness processes and the effect that their actions have on it. Better implementation of treatment may be achieved if patients are allowed to participate in the planning of their treatment. This may not only guarantee better outcomes in a process where neither physician nor patient has complete control, but may also assist in a process of learning.
- Physicians as expert planners have no moral authority as far as the condition of patients is concerned. Therefore, patients must be able to participate in planning their treatments in order to have their wishes and values included in the decision. Physicians and patients therefore both ought to be decision makers.
- Physicians control the means for implementing treatment directly (knowledge and skills) and additional resources required for treatment (hospital, medication, diagnostic equipment, and so on) indirectly. They are not in control of the health care environment described earlier (government regulations, business, and so on) that may influence their ability to use available resources.
- Physicians, as experts, have to be aware of the poverty of their knowledge. They ought to constantly reflect on what they know and how they know that to be true. Churchman's method is a powerful tool for achieving this goal. Furthermore, it ought to be their constant purpose to increase their knowledge through learning by self-reflection, communication with their colleagues, and continuous education.
- As the manager of illness, physicians ought to act ethically. There is nothing new to this, since the Oath administered to newly qualified physicians has this as its aim.
- Finally, physicians must reflect on the inability of their craft to solve in a logical way many of the problems presented to it. Their inability to do so is the reason that their "enemies", the alternative approaches, are sought out by many patients. Furthermore, it is the reason that the moral, political, and religious enemies, are attempting to control the patient-physician interaction. Their views are valid, since physicians have not shown that they can ensure improvement by acting responsibly by the use of a different approach to diagnosis and treatment.

Alternative medicine nowadays has a distinct following, because modern physicians lost the inability to listen to their patients' problems, and because of the failure of their science to "cure" in ways that patients expect. The failure is because they still rely on a linear causality model of illness that assumes they are experts and in complete control.

In sum, the application of Churchman's approach to inquiry and his method to diagnosis could significantly increase the rigor of the system, and therefore the quality of decision-making. This could lead to better quality treatment and reduced cost. The education of modern medical professionals does not equip them with such a system of inquiry and the ideal would be to introduce it as part of a revised curriculum. It could also be taught to physicians employed by government and managed care organizations.

Synthesis

What then is the potential effect of a systems model on the patient-physician system? (**Diagram 28**)

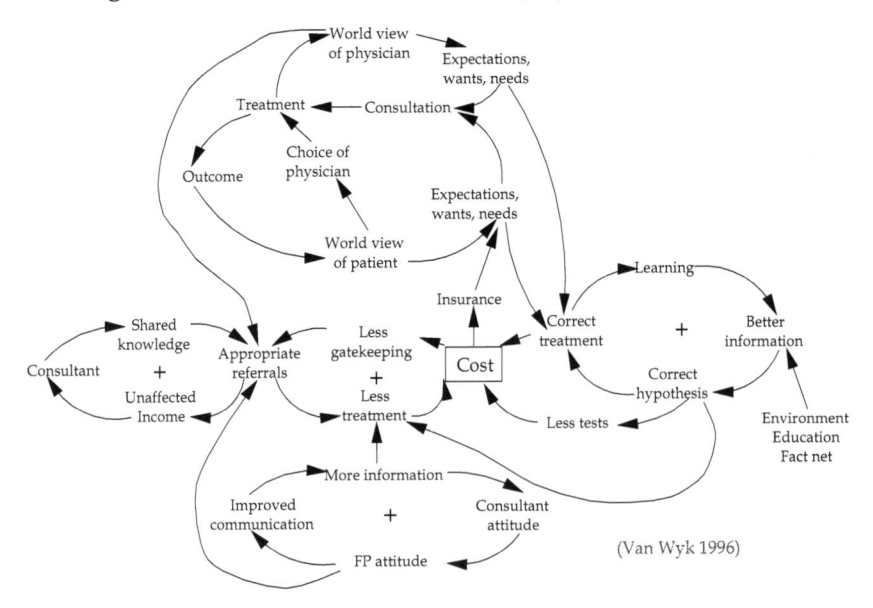

Diagram 28: Cost-effective Patient-physician Interaction

(Van Wyk 1996)

(This diagram should be read in comparison to **diagram 24**, page 199).

1. A changed worldview of health, illness and health care may help patients to learn how their wants and expectations affect the system as a whole and therefore ultimately cost. They may learn that their actions lead to increased insurance contributions or taxes and that these may be avoided by altering their behavior and map of health care. Changing the

social mind map of health care may prove to be the most powerful intervention for improving and returning stability to the system.
- An altered worldview may lead to the selection of physicians that have the ability to return patients to self care in a more efficient manner This would lead to improved treatment, better outcomes and reduced costs, and better outcomes will reinforce the new worldview. I.e. this could become a reinforcing loop and also create an indirect incentive for physicians to improve their knowledge and skills in order to contract with more patients.
- A systems model of health could lead to different wants and expectations, which affect the consultation system. A changed worldview may lead to a more efficient consultation process, better treatment, better outcomes, and so on.
- A systems view may lead to the expectation of correct and better treatments. Improved treatment will lead to reduced costs less medical insurance, and therefore a reinforcement of the worldview.

2. Physicians may learn how their actions affect the system, and that they may reduce costs by sharing responsibility, although not at their own expense.
- A changed view of their role as professionals could lead to changed expectations, wants, and needs, which affects the consultation system. A better consultation system may lead to improved treatment and outcomes, and therefore a reinforcement of the worldview. This could become a reinforcing loop that interacts synergistically with that of the patient worldview.
- The altered worldview may increase the number of appropriate referrals and therefore have a positive effect on the physician network. This could stabilize remuneration, allay uncertainties, and therefore reinforce the worldview.
- A systems view creates expectations of correct and better treatment, and leads to reduced costs.

3. The effect of a physician network that flows from the systems model of health could be threefold. These loops are connected and reinforce each other.
- Remuneration rewards the efficient use of knowledge and skills and therefore purpose. Family practitioners and consultants no longer compete for funding since they are rewarded for fulfilling different purposes. This could lead to increased sharing of knowledge and more appropriate referrals. Appropriate referrals ensure a sufficient income to consultants, who are more inclined to share knowledge and a reinforcing loop is created.
- The improved attitude of consultants could lead to an improved attitude of family practitioners, better communication, and increased sharing of clinical information. This may reinforce the positive attitude of consultants. The sharing of clinical information also leads

to less repetition in testing and prescribing, less treatment, more appropriate treatment, and less cost.
- Family practitioners no longer feel threatened by consultants, leading to more purposeful communication and more appropriate (early) referrals. This may lead to better treatment and less cost.
- Furthermore, more appropriate referrals and less treatment reduces the need for gatekeeping. This may lead to less resentment from consultants, more appropriate referrals, and so on.

4. In a systems model of health, patients and physicians would expect better and more purposeful treatment. This could improve the learning of correct methods of treatment, leading to better information and knowledge, better diagnoses, and better treatment. The latter in turn leads to reduced costs. Furthermore, better diagnoses could lead to fewer tests and therefore a further reduction in cost.
5. A reduction in cost is achieved in the patient-physician system through less and better treatment, and fewer tests. This could result in a reduced need for gatekeeping and a reduction in patient insurance.

A systems model of health may also have the following effects.

- A multiple causality model of illness may lead to a better understanding of what is achievable and how. It may lead to the more efficient use of information, an increased number of correct diagnoses, more correct treatment, and learning. The latter could feed back into more knowledge and this loop could become a positive reinforcement loop for knowledge. Furthermore, it could lead to more appropriate research that could also reinforce learning.
- A changed map of physicians may identify a different purpose for them in the health care system. They become members of a community of physicians, who in turn are part of the community as a whole. Therefore, physicians would not lose their status in society, but on the contrary, they may resume a more traditional role.
- The role of alternative medicine was defined as contributing towards and not opposing traditional health care. This may lead to better interaction between traditional and alternative healers, since both are included in the health care system as part of a dialectic synthesis.
- The application of Churchman's method to the diagnostic cycle may have a profound influence on the quality of diagnosis and decision-making. This may in turn improve the quality of treatment and reduce cost.

A systems model of health may also have an effect on the health care system on a higher level, in other words as a whole. Referring to the multiple causality model of health care (**diagram 15**, page 125), the following may happen (**diagram 29**).

Diagram 29: The Effect of the Systems Model of Health on the Mess in Health Care

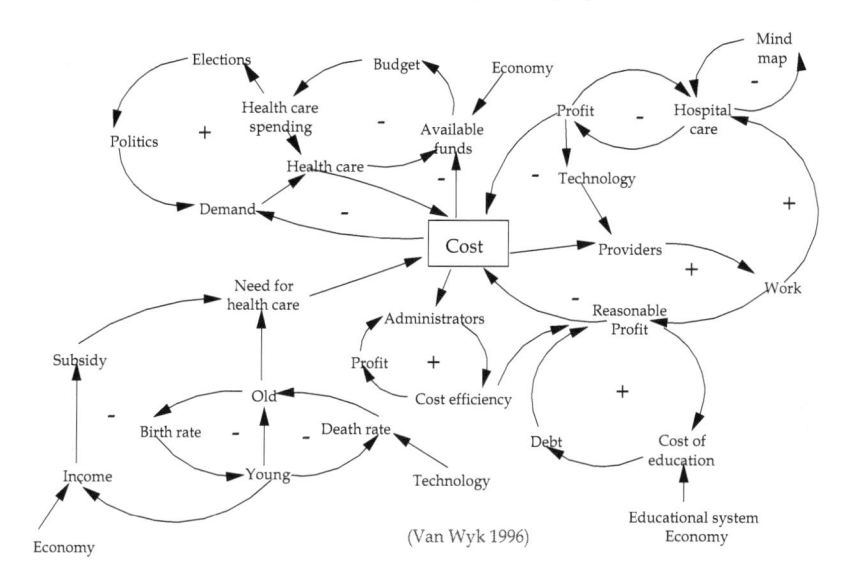

(Van Wyk 1996)

1. The systems model may have only a minor influence on the economical factors that determine the availability of health care funding, the factors that lead to an ageing population, and the power structures in the system (governments and business interests). It may have a more definitive impact on:
   - The administrator system as a profit making entity.
   - The hospital system as a profit making entity.
   - The education system, including both the medical curriculum and the cost of education to newly qualified physicians.
   - The political system and their use of health care demand to ensure electability.
   - The factors that disturb the ability of the young to cross subsidize the elderly.
   - The legal system as a profit making entity.
2. An altered worldview could alter the demand for health care. This could reduce the need for health care delivery with a lessened impact of the political loop. A decreased demand could lead to less work and less cost. This in turn could reduce the demand on the budget for health care funding.
3. The systems view of health care may question the desirability of attempts by science to discover ways for ensuring eternal life. This may alter the wants, needs, and expectations of the community, with more attention to the needs of the elderly, as opposed to wants and expectations. This may reduce the need for expensive technology and increase the application of

appropriate treatment, which in turn may reduce the cost to the system and the need for a crippling subsidy by the young.
4. An altered remuneration system may reduce the incentive for abuse and exorbitant profits. Therefore there may be less inappropriate work in the system and decreased cost. In other words, physicians may reduce their demands on the system.
- The cost of health care education is a problem of the larger environment and will need to be attended to as such. It is often stated that physicians have an obligation towards the community, because their education was subsidized by the state through taxes. This argument does not take into consideration the fact that physicians, by virtue of their income, will in turn contribute towards society by the taxes they pay. Furthermore, members of other professions, such as law, engineering, and so on appear to be exempt from this argument.
- More responsible and better treatment may lead to reduced litigation and therefore reduced malpractice insurance. This may affect the legal system. The realization that physicians are not in control of illness and health care processes (a traditional assumption) may also influence the findings of inquests into possible negligence.
- The tension between physicians and health care administrators will continue, unless the principles of a systems approach to health care could be expanded to this level. Administrators at present appear to be unwilling to explain to physicians how savings and profits in health care will benefit the system. If physicians do not feel that they will benefit from a more efficient system, they will be unwilling to implement planning to improve the system. The question of whether it is ethical to make a profit from members of the community in distress, and if so, how much is appropriate or desirable, will need to be answered as part of an inquiry into the values of the system.
5. A systems approach to health care may reduce the demand for high-technology treatment as a result of a better understanding of the relative value of it. This could reduce the amount of inappropriate work.
6. The changed worldview requires a shift away from hospital care. This will affect the profits of hospitals and eventually also the demand for high-technology treatments and research. The emphasis is on appropriate specialist care as described earlier, the purpose being to move patients back into the community as soon as possible.

In many of the systems participating in the health care system, a political metaphor is operative. Hence, it may prove in time that in spite of advantageous changes that patients and physicians may be prepared to make, gains could be lost as a result of the power plays in these systems. Therefore, the implementability of the systems model of health will in the end depend upon its environment. However, this does not imply that no attempt should be made to improve the system at grass roots level.

In summary, this chapter showed how the application of Churchman's system of inquiry and method may be used for solving the questions posed in earlier chapters. The approach was used for discovering and exploring an alternative worldview of health, illness and health care. The advantage of this worldview is that it takes a broad view of illness and health in society, and its application has implications for the purposeful components of the system. Ways to implement a systems model of health was explored and it would appear as if changing the way that patients and physicians think and interact, may have a powerful influence on the efficiency of the health care system as a whole. This may contribute towards a more affordable system. In terms of Churchman's approach, the implementation of a new worldview does not satisfy a short-term goal, its aim is to achieve a long-term ideal and is therefore an evolving learning process.

The application of Churchman's thinking to the diagnosis and treatment may improve the efficiency of decision-making. It supports the more efficient use and application of knowledge to this process, and leads to increased learning. Physicians may learn by constant reflection about their knowledge and the outcomes of their decisions, and patients through their involvement in the decision-making process.

The aim of this study was to explore the reasons why the health care system is not functioning properly. The systems approach in general and C West Churchman's general systems theory in particular, is a suitable method for answering the question how can the problems of the health care system be resolved? However, ultimately the perspective is that of a planner and does not include viewpoints that may arise from the participation in planning by other parties. To be truly systemic, these ideas must become part of purposeful social inquiry that includes the clients whose wishes are to be attended to, and the decision makers with the resources to actually implement change.

Chapter 10: The Decision Support System

Systems thinking was shown earlier to be founded on a systems philosophy (in this book Churchman's), at the next level on a wholismic perspective, or systems approach, and finally the application of a systems methodology to a real world problem (refer to **diagram 4**, page 30). The question of an appropriate methodology was deliberately avoided until now, because of the risk that the focus may become a specific method at the expense of the other two levels of systems thinking. Having placed the argument firmly on the proposed systems philosophy and worldview, this chapter is a provisional attempt at a methodology that could take the argument further and constructively assist in practical purposeful inquiry. The approach is a modification Checkland's (1991) Soft Systems Methodology (SSM) into a more comprehensive model that will be called the Decision Support System (DSS) to distinguish it from SSM proper.

Diagram30: Soft Systems Methodology

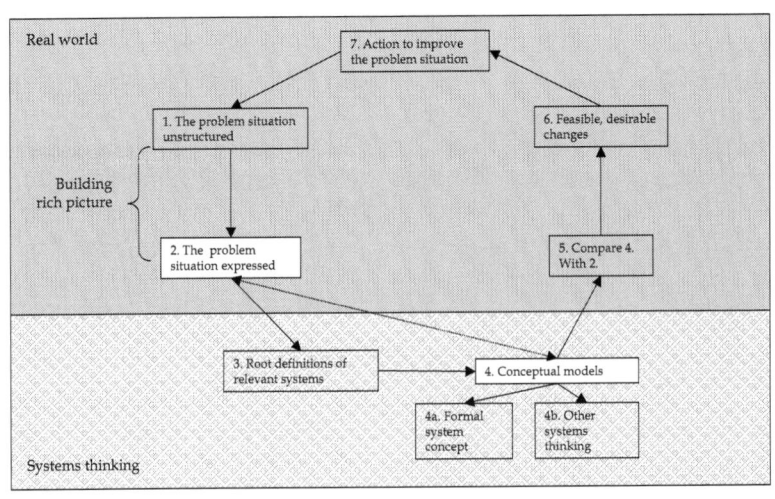

(Adapted with permission from: Checkland, P. *Systems Thinking, Systems Practice*. Copyright © 1991 John Wiley and Sons Limited)

Soft systems methodology

The history and evolution of SSM was discussed earlier, hence the focus here is on the practicalities of the model itself.

In common with all systems methodologies SSM begins by defining the problem situation, which Checkland defines as a condition characterized by a sense of mismatch that eludes precise definition between the perception of what is and what may become actuality (**diagram 30**). During the first two stages, an attempt is made to build a "rich picture" of the problem situation[1], which is similar to Ackoff's mess or problematique referred to earlier. The purpose of this stage is to consider as many perceptions about the problem situation as possible, which in terms of Churchman's methodology may suggest possible relevant solutions.

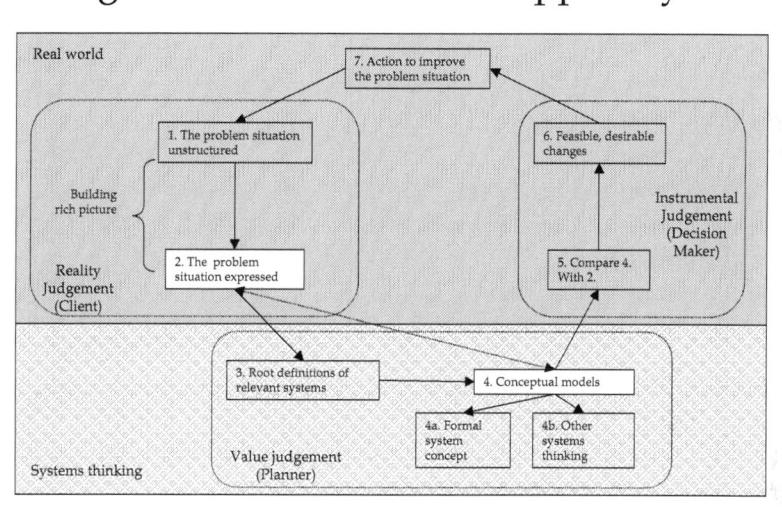

Diagram 31: The Decision Support System

During stages 3 and 4, conceptual models are designed based on a systems view of the world, which in stage 5 is compared to reality in order to generate a dialogue that may lead to feasible and desirable changes. Checkland makes a critical distinction between the real world and the notional world of systems thinking, which divides the model into the worlds of common sense and logic. Methodologically, real world inquiry requires a continuous process of discussion and dialogue between all participants, whereas logic is based on questioning, which involves inquiry and reflection. In other words, inquiry into social phenomena requires both logic and dialogue and is incomplete if the observer or planner relies on either one or the other alone.

---

[1] As opposed to the problem itself.

It is possible to enhance Checkland's SSM model by infusing into it aspects of Vickers' appreciative system model and Churchman's method of inquiry described earlier.

The Decision Support System

Appreciation

Checkland's SSM is validated by Vickers' appreciative system. Building the rich picture (stages 1 and 2) is the equivalent of the reality judgment (what is), stages 3 and 4 to the value judgment (what ought to be), and stages 5 and 6 with the instrumental judgment (what should be done)(**diagram 31**).

Churchman's inquiring system

Checkland used some of Churchman's notions about systems in the design of stages 3 and 4, but Churchman's approach potentially has a much wider application. The client is the problem owner and as such the main actor in the reality judgment, the decision maker has the resources to change the client's reality, and the planner aims to bring the two together during the value judgment. Furthermore, a critical issue of Churchman's design remains an awareness of the sources of knowledge, and the sweeping in of value and other issues. Also, in the Churchmanian system the sources of control are pervasive within the system of inquiry; therefore implementation is guaranteed by the participation of all actors in the process of inquiry.

Systems methodologies

Flood and Jackson (1991) proposed an attractive approach termed *Total Systems Intervention* (TSI) according to which the different systems methodologies may be considered as a toolbox from which the appropriate one may be selected to attack a specific problem. It is therefore just a matter of matching the appropriate methodology to the right problem. The flaw in the approach is the assumption that one methodology is relevant to one particular problem type. The approach taken here is that the argument of TSI is sound, but that different methodologies have different strengths to offer during the *process* of any inquiry as such. Hence, at different times the strengths of different methodologies are utilized to enhance the process of inquiry, thereby avoiding their inherent weaknesses that Flood and Jackson pointed out.

The basis of TSI is the division of problem situations into six categories depending on the nature of the system (closed or open) and the relationship between the people that participate in it (unitary, pluralist, or coercive)(**Table 8**). In terms of this grouping, analytical methodologies are appropriate for inquiry into closed systems with unified relationships, but for open systems with pluralist relationships, such as occur in most social systems, one of the approaches based on Churchman's philosophy is necessary.

Table 8: A Grouping of Problem Contexts

		Relationship Between Participants		
		Unitary	Pluralist	Coercive
		# Shared common interests # Compatible values & beliefs # Agreement on means & ends # Participation in decision making # Actions in accordance with agreed objectives	# Interests compatible # Some divergence of values & beliefs # Disagreement but compromise possible on means & ends # Participation in decision making # Actions in accordance with agreed objectives	# Common interests not shared # Conflicting values & beliefs # Disagreement & compromise not possible on means & ends # Coercion to accept decisions # Agreement on objectives impossible
		Systems Methodologies		
Nature of System	Simple (Closed Systems) # Small number of elements # Few interactions # Attributes predetermined # Interactions highly organized # Behaviour governed by laws # Stable over time # Parts not purposeful # Closed to environment	# Operations Research # Systems Analysis (RAND) # Systems Engineering # System Dynamics (Forrester, Kauffman, Senge)	# Strategic Assumption Surfacing and Testing (Mason & Mitroff)	# Critical Systems Heuristics (Ulrich)
	Complex (Open Systems) # Many elements # Many interactions # Attributes not predetermined # Interactions loosely organized # Probabilistic # Evolves over time # Parts purposeful # Open to environment	# Viable System Diagnosis (Beer) # General System Theory (Von Bertalanffy) # Socio-technical Systems (Tavistock)	# Interactive Planning (Ackoff) # Soft Systems Methodology (Checkland)	# None

(Adapted from Flood and Jackson (1991))

Interactive planning

Ackoff's (1981) Interactive Planning (IP) may contribute towards the DSS described here in two ways. Firstly by way assisting in formulating the mess, which applies to stages 2 and 3, and secondly, by ideals planning, which is particularly relevant for finding desirable changes to resolve the problem situation in stage 6.

Systems inquiry

Strümpfer's (1992) model for systems inquiry is currently the best available method for inquiry into complex systems, which applies to stages 3 and 4 of the DSS. This method includes System Dynamics modeling, which gives information about the process dimension of systems, and Beer's Viable System Model, which is currently the only satisfactory model for explaining the behavior of organizations from a systems perspective.

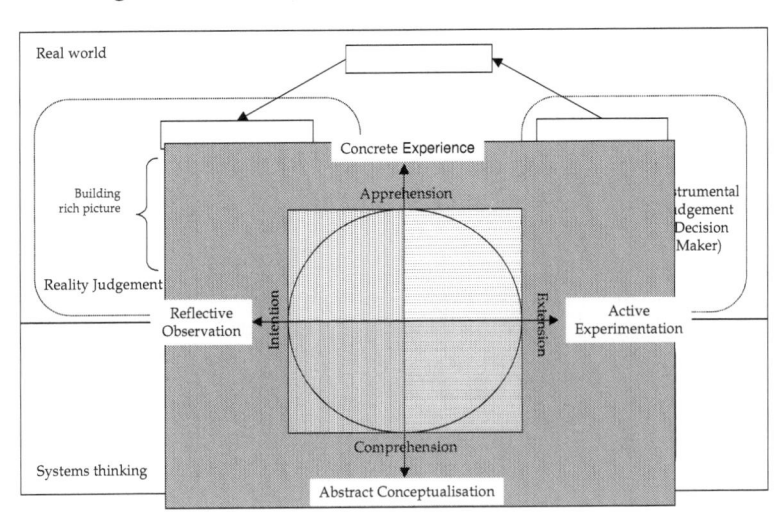

Diagram 32: Kolb's Learning Cycle and SSM

Critical Systems Heuristics

Ulrich's (1994b) is the only available methodology for addressing the problem of political planning or coercive issues. This would apply to stages 5 to 7, since in the real world change and implementation is often a process of negotiation influenced by power, cultural, and other organizational issues.

Learning

Checkland is very explicit about the fact that SSM is a learning system, in that the problem situation is transformed by inquiry into new attitudes and ways of doing things. This is in keeping with both Lewin's and Singer's notions of knowledge as a chain of problems towards which inquiry, the solution of the problem and by extension learning, contribute. Furthermore, Kolb's (1984) learning system model described earlier is super-imposable on the DSS model as follows (**diagram 32**).

The problem situation is the outcome of a feeling of discomfort about which there is reflection (stages 1 and 2). During the next phase (stage 3), theories are created by analysis and reflection, followed by model construction for the purpose of manipulating the external world (stage 4) based on logic, ending in active implementation (stages 5 to 7). If this conceptualization is accepted, Checkland's SSM is indeed a learning cycle.

Given the fact that learning and knowledge is intimately linked, Kolb's model has a definite epistemological connotation. Based on the work of the philosopher Stephen Pepper, he suggests that each of four learning styles is related to current epistemological models. These are

- Divergent knowledge with the common sense, intuitive of the cognitive approaches
- Assimilative knowledge with the logical-theoretical aspects of the rationalist tradition
- Convergent knowledge with the logical aspects of empiricism, and
- Accommodative knowledge with the purposeful action-orientated pragmatic tradition.

A complete theory of knowledge therefore needs to dialectically include all of these traditions[2]. Also, a strength of the model is that it recognizes the dialectical tension between the purely rational and purely intuitive on the one hand, and purely introspective and purely action orientation on the other. Hence, any either-or theory of knowledge at any of the extremes is incomplete, which is why each of the traditions may be criticized as indicated earlier in the text. Furthermore, any learning or inquiry based on the appropriate methodology of one tradition alone will provide incomplete knowledge. For example, based on this argument, the empirical scientific tradition is incomplete by ignoring the metaphysical issues of values, denying the influence of cognitive bias, and often also the purposeful nature of inquiry.

---

[2] This proposition implies Churchman's notion about the sources of knowledge.

Kolb's model suggests that the verification of objective truth depends on the completeness of inquiry, which although it can never be attained to perfection, can aim for the ideal of comprehensiveness. On a practical level, it means that objective truth consists of both the real world (intuition and common sense) and logic, and both phenomenal and symbolic knowledge, and that to arrive at it requires a comprehensive methodology of inquiry that recognizes this. The proposed DSS has features compatible with this ideal and satisfies Churchman's criteria for inquiry systems.

Implementation and change

From a practical perspective, stages 6 and 7 involve the real world problems of change and implementation. This in itself is a large subject, and what follows is therefore just a brief overview.

Change

According to Lewin (1997), individuals can only change relative to the group they belong to, and successful permanent change in groups requires three steps.

i. **Unfreezing**
   Pedler and Aspinwall (1998) is of the opinion that there are three criteria for successful change to occur, dissatisfaction with the status quo, a desirable alternative vision for the future, and a credible method or process for getting there. Also, the sum of the criteria must be more than the pain caused by and cost of change[3]. According to Gharajedaghi (1999), the best method for unlearning is by making assumptions explicit by public discourse and dialogue. People are more likely to understand and voluntarily participate in change if they are allowed to partake in planning change (Kreitner and Kinicki, 1992).

ii. **Change**
   According to Senge (1994; 1990), the object of group learning is to make shared images and assumptions explicit. In this way belief systems may be altered or manipulated to the advantage of the group, and he suggests that a useful method for doing so is by way of a structured dialogue[4]. Since learning is a cognitive process (Lewin, 1997), the ability to question efficiently requires reflective and inquiry skills (Senge, 1994), a deep understanding of existing beliefs[5] and a definitive outcome (or vision) to guide the process of changing perceptions.

iii. **Refreezing**
   If leaders convince a group to act based on their beliefs and if the solution works and the group shares a perception of success, then the

---

[3] $D + V + M > P$
[4] Refer here to the hermeneutic tradition.
[5] What Carnall (1999) calls cognitive capability

value judgment that the solution is "good" starts a process of cognitive transformation from a shared belief into a shared assumption or new mind map. Typically, social validation of the acceptability of the solution depends on the degree to which it reduces anxiety and is accepted.

Implementation

A systems analysis of implementation as a symbolic problem indicates that a critical issue for implementation is changing the ways people do things, or group culture, which is a regulator of human activity (Van Wyk, 2000). Culture in turn is regulated by assumptions about reality; hence to change culture, the basic beliefs, or mind maps of a group must be changed. Facilitative leadership and a clear vision for the future are critical for initiating change and changing belief systems, and the best way for changing belief systems is by action learning, during which prevailing knowledge is changed by questioning (reflection and inquiry). Participation in collective inquiry is critical for developing a shared understanding and enhances the possibility of successful implementation.

Summary

The Decision Support System is a meta-model of inquiry in the true sense of the word. It is not only grounded on a sound philosophical and rationally defendable basis, but also utilizes the full spectrum of systems methodologies. As such, it has the potential to make an important contribution to the systems debate.

No doubt, the reader will be aware by now that the DSS model was used in this text up to SSM stage 5. Consequently, the views in this book are that of a planner and their utility in practice can only be tested in the real world once they have been subjected to the scrutiny of the clients of the system. In addition, a decision maker sharing in the vision and with the resources and desire to make the plan work is a prerequisite.

Epilogue

We saw in this text that social and organizational planning depends critically on the assumptions we make about the world that we live in. We can conceive of nature and society as reasonably simple, stable and predictable, or as consisting of complex systems of numerous components and actors that influence each other all the time and that have properties that depend on how the parts interact with each other.

The former view lends itself to investigation and decision making by analysis and reduction, which represents inter alia the bulk of modern social and business planning methods. But the fact is that using the best of what these methods can offer, less than 10% of strategic plans will be implemented (Hardy, quoted in Carnall (1997b)), 60 to 80% of Business Process Reengineering projects fail to meet their objectives (Scott-Morgan quoted in Carnall (1997a)), and 75% of attempted business turnarounds fail (Slatter, quoted in Carnall (1997a)). In addition, many plans have been spectacularly unsuccessful when dealing with complex issues (see for example Hall (1980)), or have had disastrous unplanned effects (see Tenner (1996).

The alter ego of analysis is synthetic thinking, or the systems approach, which assumes a complex world of many interactions that are dynamically changing all the time, but in spite of this exhibit stability and may be understood by taking a broad perspective. In systems, cause and effect is replaced by numerous co-producers interacting with one another to fulfill higher level functions as components of larger systems, and in which traditional command and control is meaningless. This approach offers a way of inquiring into and managing the complexity before which analysis stands paralyzed.

C West Churchman designed a system of logic, which in broad terms describes the conditions for inquiry into complex phenomena. In terms of this approach, inquiry and planning itself is a social system consisting of at least three actors, namely an "expert", or planner, a decision maker that may be in a position to release resources to realize a plan or implement a solution, and people for whom plans are made, or clients, who live with the consequences of planning.

During inquiry, those who plan should constantly reflect on the sources of the knowledge they use, which may be embedded in and supported by fact nets, or were verified by experts. Both sources are founded upon assumptions, which must be vigorously questioned. Facts themselves are systems that change all the time and to reduce the risk of failure or unwanted consequences of planning, as many aspects of and perspectives about the problem situation as possible should be considered, including the ethical and moral implications of the plan. Since analysis offers no method for managing such wide-ranging inquiry, the alternative metaphor for framing inquiry is the systems view of the world.

Churchman said that in the end, logical planning and decision-making often have to bow before the reality of the irrationality of real life. In other words, sometimes the only way to change is intuitive and irrational. Questions, and change, in the end starts with leadership – someone realizing that something is wrong and that we need to do something. In this instance, the pragmatists are correct, questions and inquiry is a purposeful activity, the question is how to do so most efficiently.

Social, or human activity systems are some of the most complex systems known. They remain stable around shared norms or beliefs, which remain tacit and untested. A breakdown of stability often acts as signal for inquiry, during which underlying norms and beliefs should be tested and adjusted when needed. Critical issues to the optimal functioning of human activity systems are participation in planning, co-operation, trust, and a shared vision of the future.

The health care system grew from a simple into an enormously complex socio-technical system that has become problematic to most countries in the world. The symptoms of system stress are a cost spiral out of control, and a breakdown of trust between various participants in the system.

The application of a systems approach to the health care system suggests that a fundamental problem is the prevailing norms and beliefs in the system, and that a promising intervention would be one able to readjust processes in the system towards a map more in keeping with modern reality. Such a map is the systems view of health presented within this text, which has numerous intriguing and large-scale implications to the system as a whole and as shown, may contribute towards reestablishing stability in the system. The systems view of health by itself does not guarantee success, but it does offer a fresh and very different approach to a so far intractable problem and therefore deserves the attention of both systems thinkers and health care planners.

Finally, the design of a Decision Support System is presented that has a sound practical, pragmatic, and philosophical background, and that may aid systems practitioners and planners in inquiry, planning, and decision-making.

In the final analysis, a systems approach is a viable alternative to the current inefficient attempts to correct the imbalance in the health care system. What is lacking is leadership and a broad vision of what an ideal health care system could look like in future. This book provides such a vision, which is not only desirable and feasible, but could perhaps restore stability. What it hopes to do is stimulate the level of debate about health care to a higher level, and perhaps convince some of those with the means to affect meaningful change, i.e. decision makers, to have the courage to do the right thing, or be heroic in Churchman's terms.

Bibliography

Anonymous (1991) Health Care. *The Economist* Suppl (6 July):3-22.

Anonymous (1992) Your Patient's Expectations. *SAPM* 14, 18-20.

Anonymous (1994a) Vital Stats. Sexual Roulette. *Newsweek* August 22, 3.

Anonymous (1994b) *A National Health Plan for South Africa*, Johannesburg: ANC.

Anonymous (1996) A "servile" France? *Newsweek* January 29, 38-39.

Ackoff, R.L. (1981) *Creating The Corporate Future. Plan or Be Planned For*, New York: John Wiley & Sons.

Ackoff, R.L. (1991) *Ackoff's Fables. Irreverent Reflections on Business and Bureaucracy*, New York: John Wiley and Sons.

Ackoff, R.L. and Emery, F.E. (1972) *On Purposeful Systems*, Chicago: Aldine Atherton.

Adams, G.B., Catron, B.L. and Cook, S.D.N. (1995). Foreword to the Centenary edition of The Art of Judgement. In Vickers, G., *The art of judgement: A study of policy making*, Sage Publications, Thousand Oaks CA.

Agnew, L.R.C., Aviado, D.M., Brody, J.I., Burrows, W., Butler, R.F., Combs, C.M., Gambill, C.M., Glasser, O., Hine, M.K., Shelley, W.B. and Daly, L.W. (1965) *Dorland's Illustrated Medical Dictionary*, 24th edn. Philadelphia: W.B. Saunders Co.

Alexander, T. (1993) One Man's Tough Choices on Prostate Cancer. *Fortune* September 20, 73-81.

Allen, R.E. (1992) *The Concise Oxford Dictionary of Current English*, 8th edn. Oxford: Clarendon Press.

Anderson, W.T. (Ed.) (1996) *The Fontana Postmodernism Reader*, London: Fontana Press.

Appignanesi, R. and Garratt, C. (1995) *Postmodernism for Beginners*, Cambridge: Icon Books Ltd.

Arrow, K.J. (1963) Uncertainty and the welfare economics of medical care. *Am Econ Rev* 53, 941-973.

Bak, P. and Kan, C. (1991) Self-organized Criticality. *Scientific American* 264, 26-33.

Bylinsky, G. (1994) The New Fight Against Killer Microbes. *Fortune* September 5, 70-75.

Balint, M. (1986) The Collusion of Anonymity. In: Balint, M. (Ed.) *The Doctor, His Patient and the Illness*, 2nd edn., Edinburgh: Churchill Livingstone.

Bateson, G. (1979) *Mind and Nature. A Necessary Unity*, New York: EP Dutton.

Benade, M.M. (1992) Distribution of Health Personnel in the Republic of South Africa with Special Reference to Medical Practitioners. *SAMJ* 82, 260-263.

Benatar, S.W. (1985) A National Health Service for South Africa. *SAMJ* 68, 839

Benningfield, P. (1995) *Health Maintenance Organizations (HMO). Are they the Solution?* Presented at the 3rd Annual Corporate Health Care Conference, Johannesburg.

Benson, G.S. (1994) The Decline of Urological Education in United States Medical Schools. *J Urol* 152, 169-170.

Berne, E. (1964) *Games People Play*, London: Penguin Books.

Berne, E. (1987) *What Do You Say After You Say Hello?* London: Corgi Books.

Berwick, D.M. (1991) Controlling Variation in Health Care. A Consultation from Walter Shewhart. *Medical Care* 29, 1212-1225.

Blum, H.L. (1983) *Expanding health care horizons. From a general systems concept of health to a national health policy*, 2nd edn. Oakland, CA: Third Party Publishing Co.

Bodenheimer, T. (1996) The HMO Backlash. Righteous or Reactionary? *NEJM* 335(21):1601-1604

Botha, J.L., Bradshaw, D. and Gonin, R. (1986) How Many Doctors are Needed in South Africa by 1990? *SAMJ* 69, 250-254.

Boulding, K. (1987) *The Image. Knowledge in Life and Society*, Ann Arbor: The University of Michigan Press.

Bowler, T.D. (1981) *General Systems Thinking. Its Scope and Applicability*, New York: Elsevier North Holland.

Brook, R.H., Chassin, M.R., Fink, A., Solomon, D.H., Kosecoff, J. and Park, R.E. (1986) A method for the detailed assessment of the appropriateness of medical technologies. *Int J Tech Assess Health Care* 2, 53-63.

Brook, R.H. (1994) Appropriateness: The next frontier. *BMJ SA* 2, 344.

Brook, R.H. and Lohr, K.N. (1985) Efficacy, Effectiveness, Variations, and Quality. Boundary-crossing Research. *Medical Care* 23, 710-722.

Broomberg, J. (1990) The Impact of Fee-For-Service Reimbursement System on the Utilisation of Health Services. Part I. A Review of the Determinants of Doctor's Practice Patterns. *SAMJ* 78, 130-132.

Broomberg, J. and Price, M.R. (1990) The Impact of Fee-For-Service Reimbursement System on the Utilisation of Health Services. Part II. Comparison of Utilisation Patterns in Medical Aid Schemes and a Local Health Maintenance Organization. *SAMJ* 78, 133-136.

Buckley, W. (1967) *Sociology and Modern Systems Theory*. New Jersey: Prentice Hall Inc.

Bunker, J.P. (1970) Surgical Manpower. A Comparison of Operations and Surgeons in the United States and in England and Wales. *NEJM* 282, 135-144.

Callahan, D. (1980) Shattuck Lecture. Contemporary Medical Ethics. *NEJM* 302, 1228-1233.

Capra, F. (1991) *The Tao of Physics. An Exploration of the Parallels Between Modern Physics and Eastern Mysticism*, Hammersmith: Flamingo.

Carnall, C. (1997a) *Changing organisations for the 21st Century*, Henley-on-Thames: Henley Management College.

Carnall, C. (1997b) *Strategic Change. Managing the process*, Henley-on-Thames: Henley Management College.

Carnall, C.A. (1999) *Managing Change In Organizations*, 3rd edn. Hempstead: Prentice Hall Europe.

Chalmers, D.J. (1995) The Puzzle of Conscious Experience. *Scientific American* 273, 62-68.

Chamberlain, E.N. and Ogilvie, C. (1974) *Symptoms And Signs In Clinical Medicine. An Introduction To Medical Diagnosis*, 9th edn. Bristol: John Wright & Sons.

Charlton, B.G. (1994) Is Inequality Bad for the National Health? *Lancet* 343, 221-222.

Checkland, P. (1991) *Systems Thinking, Systems Practice*, Chichester: John Wiley and Sons.

Checkland, P. and Scholes, J. (1991) *Soft Systems Methodology in Action*, Chichester: John Wiley & Sons.

Churchman, C.W. (1968) *The Systems Approach*, New York: Dell Publishing Co. Inc.

Churchman, C.W. (1971) *The Design of Inquiring Systems*, New York: Basic Books.

Churchman, C.W. (1979) *The Systems Approach And Its Enemies*, New York: Basic Books Inc.

Churchman, C.W. (1994) Management Science - Science of Managing and Managing of Science. *Interfaces* 24, 99-110.

Churchman, C.W. and Ackoff, R.L. (1950) *Methods of Inquiry. An Introduction to Philosophy and Scientific Method*, Saint Louis: Educational Publishers Inc.

Claassen, N.J.B. and Verschoor, T. (1992) *Medical Negligence in South Africa*, Pretoria: Digma.

Cohen, J.M. and Cohen, M.J. (1971) *The Penguin Dictionary of Quotations*, Harmondsworth: Penguin.

Colborn, R.P. (1992) Can Medical Graduates Afford to Become State Medical Officers? *SAMJ* 82, 264-266.

Coopers, Theron, du Toit (1991) *Medical Association of South Africa. Report on Recommended Tariffs. Volume 1*, Pretoria: Coopers, Theron, du Toit.

Coopers, Theron, du Toit (1992) *Medical Association of South Africa. Third Evaluation Report of the New Proposed Tariff Structure*. Pretoria: Coopers, Theron, du Toit.

Coulter, A. (1992) The Interface Between Primary and Secondary Care. In: Roland, M. and Coulter, A. (Eds.) *Hospital Referrals*, Oxford: Oxford University Press.

Cowley, G. (1993) What High Tech Can't Accomplish. *Newsweek* October 4, 32-35.

Crutchfield, J.P., Farmer, J.D., Packard, N.H. and Shaw, R.S. (1986) Chaos. *Scientific American* December, 38-49.

De Beer, C. and Broomberg, J. (1990) Financing Health Care for All - Is National Health Insurance the First Step? *SAMJ* 78, 144-147.

De Geus, A.P. (1988) Planning as Learning. *HBR* 66, 70-74.

De Geus, A.P. (1994) Modelling to Predict or to Learn? In: Morecroft, J.D.W. and Sterman, J.D. (Eds.) *Modelling for Learning Organizations*, pp. xiii-xvi. Portland: Productivity Press.

De Vree, J.K. (1994) Information in nature, human behaviour, and social life. *Behavioural Science* 39, 137-168.

De Wet, J.J. (1991) *Mediese Etiek*, Pretoria: Academica.

Dickson, G. (1995). Principles of Risk Management. In: Vincent, C. (Ed.) *Clinical Risk Management*, London: BMJ Publishers.

Dodds, M.M.E. (1993) *Nolungile Clinic, Khayelitsha: A potential model for community health care*. Research paper, University of Stellenbosch, Institute for Futures Research.

Donaldson, L.J. (1992) Maintaining Excellence. The Preservation and Development of Specialised Services. *BMJ* 305, 1280-1284.

Dooley, J. (1993) Piaget, self-organising knowledge, and critical systems practice. *Systems Practice* 6, 359-381.

Dudley, P. (1996) (Ed.) *Bogdanov's Tektology. Book 1*, Centre for Systems Studies: Hull.

Eddy, D.M. (1990a) Clinical Decision-making: From Theory to Practice. Anatomy of a Decision. *JAMA* 263, 441-443.

Eddy, D.M. (1990b) Clinical Decision-making: From Theory to Practice. Practice Policies - What are They? *JAMA* 263, 877-880.

Eddy, D.M. (1990c) Clinical Decision-making: From Theory to Practice. The Challenge. *JAMA* 263, 287-290.

Editorial (1993) Drug Promotion. Stealth, Wealth and Safety. *Lancet* 341, 1507-1508.

Editorial (1995) Sounding the Death Knell for Generalists. *Hosp Update* 5, 4

Engelhardt, H.T. and Rie, M.A. (1988) Morality for the Medical-industrial Complex. A Code of Ethics for the Mass Marketing of Health Care. *NEJM* 319, 1086-1089.

Faltermayer, E. (1994) How to Disarm Health Care's Hidden Bomb. *Fortune* 130, 88-91.

Faure, M. and Venter, A. (1993) Karl Popper's critical rationalism. In: Snyman, J. (Ed.) *Conceptions of Social Inquiry*, Pretoria: HSRC.

Feinstein, A.R. (1988) Fraud, distortion, delusion, and consensus: The problems of human and natural deception in epidemiologic science. *Am J Med* 84, 475-478.

Fitzpatrick, J.M., Dreikorn, K., Khoury, S., Koyanai, T. and Perrin, P. (1991) The Medical Management of BPH with Agents other than Hormones or alpha-blockers. In: *Proceedings. The International Consultation on Benign Prostatic Hypertrophy 1991*, London: Scientific Communication International Ltd.

Flood, R.L. and Jackson, M.C. (1991) *Creative Problem Solving. Total Systems Intervention*, Chichester: John Wiley and Sons.

Forrow, L., Taylor, W.C. and Arnold, R.M. (1992) Absolutely Relative: How Research Results are Summarised can Affect Treatment Decisions. *Am J Med* 92, 121-124.

Frankel, S. (1991) Health Needs, Health-care Requirements, and the Myth of Infinite Demand. *Lancet* 337, 1588-1590.

Fryer, G.E., Green, L.A., Dovey, S.M., Yawn, B.P., Phillips, R.L., and Lanier, D. (2003) Variation in the Ecology of Medical Care. *Ann Fam Med* 1, 81-89.

Fuchs, V.R. (1984) The "Rationing" of Medical Care. *NEJM* 311, 1572-1573.

Garattini, S. (1997) Editorial. Financial Interests Constrain Drug Development. *Science* 275:287.

Gharajedaghi, J. (1999) *Systems Thinking. Managing chaos and complexity. A platform for designing business architecture*, Boston: Butterworth Heinemann.

Gillon, R. (1985) An Introduction to Philosophical Medical Ethics : The Arthur Case. *BMJ* 290, 1117-1119.

Glaser, W. (1993) The Competition Vogue and its Outcome. *Lancet* 341, 805-811.

Gleick, J. (1987) *Chaos. Making A New Science*, New York: Penguin Books.

Goldberger, A.L., Rigney, D.R. and West, B.J. (1990) Chaos and Fractals in Human Physiology. *Scientific American* February, 35-41.

Grant, I.N. and Dixon, A.S. (1987) "Thank you for Seeing this Patient": Studying the Quality of Communication between Physicians. *Can Fam Physician* 33, 605-611.

Grove, A. (1996) Taking on Prostate Cancer. *Fortune* May 13, 33-44.

Gruca, T.S. and Nath, D. (1994) Regulatory Change, Constraints on Adaptation and Organisational Failure. An Empirical Analysis of Acute Care Hospitals. *Strategic Management Journal* 15, 345-363.

Grumet, G.W. (1989) Health Care Rationing through Inconvenience. *NEJM* 321, 607-611.

Haeger, K. (1988) *The Illustrated History of Surgery*, Harold Starke: London.

Hall, P (1980) *Great Planning Disasters*, University of California Press: Berkeley.

Harari, O. (1995) Good/Bad News About Strategy. *Management Review* July, 29-31.

Hemenway, D., Killen, A., Cashman, S., B, Parks, C.L. and Bicknell, W.J. (1990) Physician's Response to Financial Incentives. Evidence from a For-profit Ambulatory Care Center. *NEJM* 322, 1059-1063.

Hillman, A.L., Pauly, M.V. and Kerstein, J.J. (1989) How do Financial Incentives Affect Physician's Clinical Decisions and the Financial Performance of Health Maintenance Organizations? *NEJM* 321, 86-92.

Hillman, A.L., Welch, P. and Pauly, M.V. (1992) Contractual Arrangements Between HMO's and Primary Care Physicians. *Medical Care* 30, 136-148.

Hollingdale, R.J. (1966) *Western Philosophy. An Introduction*, London: Kahn & Averill.

Holtgrewe, H.L. (1993) Our Nation's Health Care Dilemma: Who Pays, How do We Pay, What Can We Afford? *J Urol* 150, 303-309.

Hookway, C. (1985) *Peirce*, London: Routledge & Kegan Paul.

Hupkes, G.J. (1992) Health Economics. *SAPM* 11, 28-39.

Hutch, J.A. and Rambo, O.N. (1970) A study of the anatomy of the prostate, prostatic urethra and the urinary sphincter system. *J Urol* 104, 443-452.

Iglehart, J.K. (1986) Canada's Health Care System (First of Three Parts). *NEJM* 315, 202-208.

Iglehart, J.K. (1991) Germany's Health Care System (First of Two Parts). *NEJM* 324, 503-508.

Iglehart, J.K. (1992a) The American Health Care System. Medicare. *NEJM* 327, 1467-1472.

Iglehart, J.K. (1992b) The American Health Care System. Managed Care. *NEJM* 327, 742-747.

Illich, I. (1976) *Medical Nemesis. The Expropriation of Health*, Pantheon Books: New York.

Jackson, M.C. (1991) The Origins and Nature of Critical Systems Thinking. *Systems Practice* 4, 131-149.

Kaplan, H.I. and Sadock, B.J. (1991) *Synopsis of Psychiatry*, 6th edn. Baltimore: Williams & Wilkins.

Kass, L.R. (1983) Professing Ethically. On the Place of Ethics in Defining Medicine. *JAMA* 249, 1305-1310.

Kauffman, D. (1980) *Systems I: An Introduction to Systems Thinking*, Minneapolis: Future Systems.

Kauffman, S.A. (1991) Antichaos and Adaptation. *Scientific American* 265, 64-70.

Kingman, S. (1994) Quality Control for Medicine. *New Scientist* 143, 22-26.

Kirton, M. (1989) A Theory of Cognitive Style. In: Kirton, M. (Ed.) *Adaptors and Innovators. Styles of Creativity and Problem Solving*, London: Routledge.

Knowles, J.H. (1973) The Hospital. *Scientific American* 229 (September), 128-137.

Kock, N.F., McQueen, R.J. and Baker, M. (1996) Learning and process improvement in knowledge organizations: A critical analysis of four contemporary myths. *The Learning Organization* 3, 31-41.

Kolb, D.A. (1984) *Experiential Learning. Experience as the Source of Learning and Development*, Englewood Cliffs: Prentice Hall.

Kongstvedt, P.R. (1989) Negotiating and Contracting with Consultants. In: Kongstvedt, P.R. (Ed.) *The Managed Health Care Handbook*, Gaithersburg: Aspen Publishers Inc.

Kreitner, R. and Kinicki, A. (1992) *Organizational behavior*, 2nd edn. Homewood, Il: Irwin.

Kriel, J. (1996) How Medicine lost Consciousness. *SA Family Practice*, 361-366.

Kronick, R., Goodman, D.C., Wennberg, J.E. and Wagner, E. (1993) The Marketplace in Health Reform. The Demographic Limitations of Managed Competition. *NEJM* 328, 148-152.

Kuhn, T.S. (1962) *The Structure of Scientific Revolutions*, Chicago: Univ of Chicago Press.

Kunin, C.M. (1987) *Detection, Prevention and Management of Urinary Tract Infections*, 4th edn. Philadelphia: Lea & Febiger.

Kvale, S. (1996) Themes of Postmodernity. In: Anderson, W.T. (Ed.) *The Fontana Postmodernism Reader*, pp. 18-25. London: Fontana Press.

Labrie, F. (1993) Intracrinology. Its Impact on Prostate Cancer. *Current Opinion In Urology* 3, 381-387.

Laffel, G. and Blumenthal, D. (1989) The Case for Using Industrial Quality Management Science in Health Care Organizations. *JAMA* 262, 2869-2873.

Lawrence, M. (1993) What is Medical Audit? In: Lawrence, M. and Schofield, T. (Eds.) *Medical Audit in Primary Health Care*, Oxford: Oxford University Press.

Leape, L. (1994). The Preventability of Medical Injury. In: Bogner, M.S (Ed.). *Human Error in Medicine*, Hove: Lawrence Erlbaum Associates.

Leutwyler, K. (1995) The price of prevention. *Scientific American* April, 96-103.

Levey, S. and Hesse, D.D. (1985) Bottom-line Health Care? *NEJM* 312, 644-647.

Levinsky, N.G. (1984a) Learning to say "No". *NEJM* 311, 1569-1575.

Levinsky, N.G. (1984b) The Doctor's Master. *NEJM* 311, 1573-1575.

Lewin, K. (1997) *Resolving social conflicts and field theory in social science*, Washington DC: American Psychological Association.

Linstone, H.A. and Mitroff, I.I. (1994) *The Challenge of the 21st Century. Managing Technology and Ourselves in a Shrinking World.* New York: State University of New York Press.

Logie, D. (1993) Zimbabwe: Health or Debt. *Lancet* 341, 950

Lomas, J., Enkin, M., Anderson, G.M., Hannah, W.J., Vayda, E. and Singer, J. (1991) Opinion Leaders vs. Audit and Feedback to Implement Practice Guidelines. Delivery after Previous Caesarean Section. *JAMA* 265, 2202-2207.

Lowsley, O.S. (1912) The Development of the human prostate gland with reference to the development of other structures at the neck of the urinary bladder. *Am J Anat* 13, 299

Luft, H.S. (1978) How do Health Maintenance Organizations Achieve their "Savings"? *NEJM* 298, 1336-1343.

Manganyi, N.C., Marais, H.C., Mauer, K.F. and Prinsloo, R.J. (1993) *Dissident Amongst Patriots*, Pretoria: HSRC.

Marwick, C. (1992) Using High-Quality Providers to Cope with Today's Rising Health Care Costs. *JAMA* 268, 2142-2145.

Maslow, A.H. (1968) *Toward A Psychology Of Being*, 2nd edn. New York: Van Nostrand Reinhold Co.

Mbiti, J.S. (1971) *African Religions and Philosophy*, London: Heinemann.

McIntyre, N. and Popper, K. (1983) The Critical Attitude in Medicine. The Need for a New Ethics. *BMJ* 287, 1919-1923.

McNeal, J.E. (1972) The Prostate and prostatic urethra: a morphologic synthesis. *J Urol* 107, 1008-1016.

McNeil, B.J., Pauker, S.G., Sox, H.C. and Tversky, A. (1982) On the elicitation of preferences for alternative therapies. *NEJM* 306, 1259-1262.

McWhinney, I.R. (1989) *A Textbook of Family Medicine*, New York: Oxford University Press.

Miller, J.G. (1978) *Living Systems*, New York: McGraw Hill Book Company.

Mills, D.H. and Von Bolschwing, G.E. (1995). Clinical risk management: experiences from the United States. In: Vincent, C. (Ed.) *Clinical Risk Management*, London: BMJ Publishers.

Milstein, A., Bergthold, L. and Selbovitz, L. (1989) Utilisation Review Techniques. In Pursuit of Value: American Utilisation Management at the Fifteen-year Mark. In: Kongstvedt, P.R. (Ed.) *The Managed Health Care Handbook*, Gaithersburg: Aspen Publishers Inc.

Mitroff, I.I and Linstone, H.A. (1993) *The Unbounded Mind. Breaking the Chains of Traditional Business Thinking*. New York: Oxford University Press.

Moray, N. (1994) Error Reduction as a Systems Problem. In: Bogner, M.S. (Ed.) *Human Error in Medicine*, Hove: Lawrence Erlbaum Associates.

Moss, F. (1995) Risk Management and Quality of Care. In: Vincent, C. (Ed.) *Clinical Risk Management*, London: BMJ: Publications.

Mundell, I. (1992) Clinical Research Damaged by UK Health Service Reforms. *Nature* 357, 617

Naylor, C.D., Chen, E. and Strauss, B. (1992) Measured Enthusiasm. Does the Method of Reporting Trial Results Alter Perceptions of Therapeutic Effectiveness? *Ann Intern Med* 117, 916-921.

Nienaber, W. (1995) *The Doctors Take the Initiative*. Presented at the 3rd Annual Corporate Health Care Conference, Johannesburg.

Nilsson, M. (1993) Sweden's Health reform. *Lancet* 342, 979.

Patching, D. (1990) *Practical Soft Systems Analysis*, London: Pitman Publishing.

Pedler, M. and Aspinwall, K. (1998) *A concise guide to the learning organization*, London: Lemos & Crane.

Pellegrino, E.D. (1976) Medical Ethics, Education and the Physician's Image. *JAMA* 235, 1043-1044.

Pellegrino, E.D. (1987) Altruism, Self-interest and Medical Ethics. *JAMA* 258, 1939-1940.

Pistorius, G.J. and Pistorius, C.W.I. (1986) *Praktykvoering vir die Huisarts*, Pretoria: HAUM.

Price, M.R. and Broomberg, J. (1990) The Impact of Fee-For-Service Reimbursement System on the Utilization of Health Services. Part III. A Comparison of Caesarean Section Rates in White Nulliparous Women in the Private and Public Sectors. *SAMJ* 78, 136-138.

Ragg, M. (1993) Australia: Doctors threaten to walk out. *Lancet* 341, 1015-1016.

Rakel, R.E. (1990) Use of Consultants. In: Rakel, R.E. (Ed.) *A Textbook of Family Medicine*, 4th edn. Philadelphia: WB Saunders Co.

Reason, J. (1990) *Human Error*, Cambridge: Cambridge University Press.

Rothman, D.J. (1997) *Beginnings count. The technological imperative of unintended consequences*, New York: Oxford University Press.

Rovin, S., Jeharajah, N., Dundon, M.W., Bright, S., Wilson, D.H., Magidson, J. and Ackoff, R.L. (1994) *An idealized design of the U.S. health care system*, Bala Cynwyd, PA: Interact.

Runes, D.D. (1963) *Dictionary of Philosophy*, New Jersey: Littlefield Adams & Co.

Russell, B. (1993) *History of Western Philosophy*, London: Routledge.

Rutstein, D.D., Berenberg, W., Chalmers, T.C., Child, C.G., Fishman, A.P. and Perrin, E.B. (1976) Measuring the Quality of Medical Care. A Clinical Method. *NEJM* 294, 582-588.

Samuelson, R.J. (1993) Health Care. How we got into this Mess. *Newsweek* October 4, 21-24.

Saward, E.W. (1973) The Organization of Medical Care. *Scientific American* 229 (September), 169-175.

Schwartz, W.B. and Aaron, H.J. (1984) Rationing Hospital Care. Lessons from Britain. *NEJM* 310, 52-56.

Scott, H.D. and Shapiro, H.B. (1992) Universal Insurance for American Health Care. A Proposal of the American College of Physicians. *Ann Intern Med* 117, 511-519.

Senge, P.M. (1990) *The Fifth Discipline*, New York: Doubleday.

Senge, P.M., Roberts, C., Ross, R.B., Smith, B.J. and Kleiner, A. (1994) *The Fifth Discipline Fieldbook*, New York: Doubleday.

Shisana, O. and Versfeld, P. (1993) Community Participation in Health Service Institutions. *SAMJ* 83, 5-8.

Singer, C. (1961) History of Medicine. In: Ashmore, H., Dodge, J.V., Armitage, J. and Kasch, H.E. (Eds.) *Encyclopaedia Britannica. A New Survey of Universal Knowledge*, Chicago: Encyclopaedia Brittanica Ltd.

Smith, G.D. and Egger, M. (1994) Who Benefits from Medical Interventions? Treating low Risk Patients can be a High Risk Strategy. *BMJ SA* 343, 345-346.

Smith, M.J. (1989) *When I Say No, I Feel Guilty*, New York: Bantam Books.

Stacey, R. (1992) *Managing Chaos. Dynamic Business Strategies in an Unpredictable World*, London: Kogan Page Ltd.

Stimmel, B. (1992) The Crisis in Primary Care and the Role of Medical Schools. *JAMA* 268, 2060-2065.

Stix, G. (1994) The Speed of Write. *Scientific American* 271, 72-77.

Strümpfer, J.P. (1992) *Modes of Inquiry: Acquiring Knowledge About Complex Phenomena*. Working Paper. Institute for Futures Research, University of Stellenbosch.

Strümpfer, J.P. (1994a) *Participation in Management*. Presented at the South African Institute for Management Scientists Conference, Cape Town.

Strümpfer, J.P. (1994b) *Management Seminar Series*. Seminar 5. Program for Systems Management, University of Cape Town.

Taber, G.M. (1995) Remaking an Industry. *Time* September 4, 34-35.

Tarnas, R. (1991) *The Passion of the Western Mind. Understanding the Ideas that have Shaped Our World*, New York: Ballantyne Books.

Teisberg, E.O. and Porter, M.E. (1994) Making Competition in Health Care Work. *HBR* 131-141.

Tenner, E (1996) *Why Things Bite Back. Technology and the Revenge of Unintended Consequences*, Alfred a Knopf: New York.

Toffler, A. (1990) *Powershift. Knowledge, Wealth and Violence at the Edge of the 21st Century*, New York: Bantam Books.

Torbert, W.R. (1991) *The Power of Balance. Transforming Self, Society and Scientific Inquiry*, London: Sage Publications.

Tracy, L. (1995) Guest Editorial. A Map of Purposeful Behaviour. *Systems Practice* 8, 5-17.

Tuffs, A. (1993) Germany: Hitch in Medical Education reform. *Lancet* 341, 1206

Tversky, A. and Kahneman, D. (1974) Judgment Under Uncertainty: Heuristics and Biases. *Science* 185, 1124-1131.

Tversky, A. and Kahneman, D. (1981) The Framing of Decisions and the Psychology of Choice. *Science* 211, 453-458.

Ulrich, W. (1988) Guest Editorial. C West Churchman - 75 Years. *Systems Practice* 1, 341-350.

Ulrich, W. (1994a) Can We Secure Future-Responsive Management through Systems Thinking and Design? *Interfaces* 24, 26-37.

Ulrich, W. (1994b) *Critical Heuristics of Social Planning. A New Approach to Practical Philosophy*, Chichester: John Wiley & Sons.

Van Cott, H. (1994). Human Errors: Their Causes and Reduction. In: Bogner, M.S. (Ed.) *Human Error in Medicine*, Hove: Lawrence Erlbaum Associates.

Van der Molen, P.P. (1989) Adaptation-innovation and Changes in Social Structure: On the Anatomy of Catastrophe. In: Kirton, M. (Ed.) *Adaptors and Innovators. Styles of Creativity and Problem Solving*, London: Routledge.

Van Rensburg, H.C.J. and Fourie, A. (1993) Inequalities in South African Health Care. Part II. Setting the Record Straight. *SAMJ* 84, 99-103.

Van Rensburg, H.C.J. and Fourie, A. (1994) Inequalities in South African Health Care. Part I. The Problem -Manifestations and Origins. *SAMJ* 84, 95-99.

Van Wyk, G.C.B. (1996) *Medicine and medical process as a learning system*, M Phil Dissertation, University of Cape Town.

Van Wyk, G.C.B. (2000) *A systems approach to organizational culture. The key to the implementation problem?* Unpublished research paper.

Van Wyk, G.C.B. (2001) *A failed change initiative. Lessons from a personal experience*, MBA Dissertation, Henley Management College.

Vickers, G. (1968) *Value Systems and Social Process*, London: Tavistock Publications.

Vickers, G. (1969) Medicine's Contribution to Culture. In: Poynter, F.N.L. (Ed.) *Medicine and Culture*, London: FNL Wellcome Historical Medical Library.

Vickers, G. (1972) *Freedom in a Rocking Boat. Changing Values in an Unstable Society*, London: Allen Lane, The Penguin Press.

Vickers, G. (1980) *Responsibility. Its Sources and Limits*, Intersystems Publications.

Vickers, G. (1984) *The Vickers Papers*. Open Systems Group. (Ed.), London: Harper & Row.

Von Bertalanffy, L. (1968) *General System Theory. Foundations, Development, Applications*, New York: George Braziller.

Wack, P. (1985) Scenarios: uncharted waters ahead. *HBR* 63, 73-89.

Waldrop, M.M. (1992) *Complexity. The Emerging Science at the Edge of Order and Chaos*, London: Penguin Books.

Wallerstein, E. (1985) Circumcision. The Uniquely American Medical Enigma. *Urol Cl NA* 12, 123-132.

Watts, A. (1975) *Tao: The Watercourse Way*, London: Arkana.

Weed, L.L. (1968) Medical Records that Guide and Teach. *NEJM* 278, 652-657.

Wennberg, J.E. (1986) Which Rate is Right? *NEJM* 314, 310-311.

Wennberg, J.E., Freeman, J.L., Shelton, R.M. and Bubolz, T.A. (1989) Hospital Use and Mortality among Medicare Beneficiaries in Boston and New Haven. *NEJM* 321, 1168-1173.

Wennberg, J.E. (1990) Outcomes Research, Cost Containment, and the Fear of Health Care Rationing. *NEJM* 323, 1202-1204.

White, K.L., Williams, T.F. and Greenberg, B.G. (1961) The ecology of medical care. *NEJM*, 265, 885-892.

Wilson, C. (1967) *The Outsider*, London: Picador.

Winter, D.G. (1973) *The Power Motive*, New York: The Free Press.

Wiswell, T.E. (1992) Prepuce presence portends prevalence of potentially perilous periurethral pathogens. *J Urol* 148, 739-742.

Woolhandler, S. and Himmelstein, D.U. (1991) The Deteriorating Administrative Efficiency of the US Health Care System. *NEJM* 324, 1253-1258.

Index

A

a priori, 51, 58
Adverse events, 85
Agreement, 56
aligned self-control, 37
Alignment, 29
analysis, 3, 15
Appreciation, 23, 153
appreciative system, 153
assumptions, 44, 58
audit, 85
authority, 36
autonomy, 26

B

betterment, 62
Blum, 89
   definition of health, 103
Boundary, 69

C

Cartesian system, 3, 7
causality
   circular, 30
   linear, 30
   producer-product, 32
Churchman, 7, 10, 34, 128, 145, 153
client, 35, 67
complex systems, 4
complexity, 12
Comprehensiveness, 63
constraint, 18
consultation system, 106
control, 19, 29, 29, 65
co-operation, 22
creative styles, 36
critical systems heuristics, 11, 34, 155
critical systems thinking, 12
critical theory, 7

cultural barriers, 28
cybernetic thinking, 3
cybernetics, 8, 22

D

decision maker, 35, 55, 66, 68
Decision Support System, 153
decision taker, 35
deduction, 50
Democratic consensus, 38
Descartes, 3, 7, 50
diagnosis, 95, 112
diagnosis-treatment system
   Churchmanian approach, 145
diagnostic cycle, 113, 145
   knowledge, 115
diagnostic system, 74, 112
Dialectic, 59

E

economic man, 25, 26, 27
Efficiency, 142
emancipation, 26
emergence, 15, 17
empiricism, 7, 51
Endoscopy, 121
enemies of the systems approach, 64
entropy, 18
environmental fallacy, 63
equifinality, 18
equilibration, 18
Equilibrium, 18
Error in decision-making, 147
ethics, 60, 64, 70
   social, 70
experts, 60

F

Fact nets, 56, 44
feedback, 8

fee-for-service, 78
first law of thermodynamics, 18
Function, 19

G

gatekeeping, 120, 119
general systems theory, 8
government intervention, 87
Government, 86, 142
group dialogue, 44
group learning, 43
Grouping of Problem Contexts, 154
guarantor, 51, 58

H

Habermas, 7
hard systems, 9, 15, 25, 28, 68, 64
health, 98
  definition, 98
health care
  ageing population, 79
  budgetary constraints, 76
  cost, 82
  failure, 76
  interventions, 83
  over supply, 77
  private sector model, 77
  regulation, 87
  social sciences, 87
  social-insurance model, 77
  specialists, 96
  specialization, 92
  systems sciences, 89
  technology, 78
  unlimited demand, 78
Health care
  definition, 74
health care system, 75, 98
  Churchman's methodology, 138
  clients, 138
  decision maker, 141
  participation, 140
  planners, 140
  purposeful system, 132
  remuneration, 143
  systems philosophy, 143

Hegel, 7, 52, 59
Heisenberg's Law, 4
heroism, 70
hierarchy, 17
hospital, 96
hospital system, 97
Human activity systems, 23
human error, 45
  health care, 86
  laboratory testing, 121

I

ideals planning, 69, 132
illness, 108
  complex causality, 108
  deprivation model, 108
  linear cause-effect, 109
Implementation, 68, 124, 156, 157
induction, 51
information network, 136
inquiry, 54
interactive planning, 11, 155

K

Kant, 7, 30, 34, 37, 51, 58, 65
knowledge systems, 40

L

learn, 39
Learning, 39, 41
learning organization, 11
learning system, 65, 155
living systems, 15, 22
living systems theory, 9
logic, 48
Logical positivism, 52

M

Machine thinking, 3
Managed Care, 84
management science, 3, 64, 65
  health care, 84
manager, 3
Measurement, 63
mechanismic systems, 28

Medical ethics, 144
medical insurance, 97
medical knowledge
  community of experts, 117
  fact nets, 116
medical practitioners
  values, 97
medical profession, 87
Medicine
  definition, 74
mess, 76
Mind maps, 39, 42
Models of organization, 28
Modes of inquiry, 21
Morals, 70

N

negentropy, 18
Newtonian system, 3
NHS system, 77, 86, 145
non-linear systems, 12, 65, 68
non-relativistic pragmatism, 53
non-traditional medicine, 136

O

objectivity, 59
Observations, 59
ontological proof, 51
operational research, 9
organismic systems, 28, 29
organization as a social system, 29
outcomes measurements, 137

P

participation, 18, 29, 37, 69
patient
  definition, 106
  expectations, 106
  selection of family practitioners, 108
patient-physician interaction, 103
  history, 92
patient-physician system, 74
  definition, 74, 103
  learning system, 128

objective, 134
Patients, 134
pharmaceutical companies, 97
pharmaceutical industry, 117, 123
physical examination, 95
physician, 101
  control, 124
  definition, 110
  purpose, 134
  role, 110
physician network system, 135
planner, 35, 55, 66, 68, 71
polarity, 18
polis, 32, 36
political metaphor, 29
positivism, 7
postmodern, 5
power
  definition, 32
  dimensions, 36
  types, 33
power relationships, 32
pragmatism, 7, 52
prevalence of illness, 129
problem situation
  definition, 152
Process, 18
professional, 102
Progress, 60
purpose, 70
  health care system, 74
Purposeful Behavior, 38
purposeful design, 54

Q

Quality Management, 84

R

Rationalism, 7, 50
Reality judgments, 23
Reason, 38
referral, 120
referral system, 135
regulation, 24
relations, 18
Representativeness, 58

responsibility, 26, 68
Responsible, 68
rich picture, 152
risk management, 85

S

salutogenesis, 19
Scenarios, 42
schemata, 45
science, 3, 4, 30, 56, 65
Science, 7
script, 109
second law of thermodynamics, 18
self-control, 29
self-organize, 12
self-organizing systems, 8
self-regulation, 8, 15, 25
Singer, 7, 34, 53, 61, 63, 70
Social Control, 27
Social order, 24
social system metaphor, 132
social systems, 23, 65
soft systems, 9, 25
soft systems methodology, 10, 67, 152
Specialist
   definition, 118
specialist referral system, 118
   features, 119
   purpose, 119
specialization, 22, 26
stability, 19, 23
standard, 60
statistics, 3
Strategic assumption surfacing and testing, 11
Structure, 17
sweeping-in, 61
synthesis, 15
system
   definition, 15
System dynamics, 11, 19, 31
   mess in health care, 79
   model of health, 100
Systems, 54
systems analysis, 9
systems approach, 8, 69
   health care, 128
systems engineering, 9
Systems inquiry, 155
systems model of health, 129, 132, 135, 141
   clients, 139
   interpretation, 132
systems thinking, 8

T

total systems intervention, 12, 34, 155
tragedy of the commons, 25
Treatment
   decision-making, 122
trust, 26
Truth, 65

U

unstable systems, 8

V

Viable system diagnosis, 11
Vickers, 19, 23, 37
   model of health care, 131
vision, 29

W

wholismic thinking, 13
"wisdom", 20
Worldview, 60, 63, 65, 98

ISBN 1-41201390-9

Printed in Great Britain
by Amazon.co.uk, Ltd.,
Marston Gate.